DATE DUE

DEMCO 38-296

CRASH INJURIES:

How and Why They Happen

A PRIMER
For Anyone Who Cares About People in Cars

By:

Alvin S. Hyde, Ph.D., M.D.

Illustrated By:

Caitlin B. Hyde

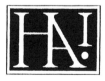

HYDE ASSOCIATES, INC.
Key Biscayne, Florida

CRASH INJURIES:

How and Why They Happen

This publication is designed to provide accurate information in regard to the subject matter covered. It is sold with the understanding that neither the author nor the publisher is engaged in the active practice of law or medicine. If legal, medical or other expert assistance is required, the services of a professional person should be sought.

From a Declaration of Principles jointly adopted by a Committee of the American Bar Association and a Committee of Publishers.

Publisher: HAI, P.O. Box 490034, Key Biscayne, Florida 33149
Compositor/Printer: P.M. Publishing & Typographics, Inc.
Typeface: 12/14 English Times

Library of Congress Cataloging-in-Publication Data

Hyde, Alvin S.

    Crash Injuries: How and Why They Happen / A Primer for Anyone Who Cares About People in Cars / Alvin S. Hyde.

    p. cm.

    ISBN   0-9637057-0-9

    1. Technical. I. Title

CONTENTS

ILLUSTRATIONS

DEDICATION AND PREFACE

I have never met Dr. Jacob Kulowski, but this book is gratefully dedicated to him.

He wrote "Crash Injuries" (Charles C Thomas, Springfield, Illinois, 1960) while in active medical practice as an orthopedic surgeon in St. Joseph, Missouri. I read it in 1961, as a research medical officer and Flight Surgeon at the Aerospace Medical Research Laboratories at Wright-Patterson Air Force Base, where I was deeply involved with how accelerative forces caused injuries and how such injuries could best be prevented.

It was the first book I had found that covered such topics both clinically and, to a useful extent, biomechanically. It seemed as if it was written just for me. In fact, it was written "primarily for physicians," dealing with "the why of automobile accidents, the how of injuries, and methods of human salvage." In some 1,080 pages, this ambitious book did just what it said it would do.

It proved to be not only useful, but to a large extent it redirected what I did and where I went within my profession for many of the years that followed.

And a lot happened in the more than 30 years that followed. For one thing, many were injured and many have died in car crashes since then. How many? Why, about 10.5 million "moderate to severe injuries" happened. And about 1.5 million killings happened. That's the equivalent, as I see it, of seriously injuring or crippling every man, woman, and child in Ohio, and then going out and slaughtering the entire living populations of Maine and Alaska.

During these past 3 decades of mutilation and killing, I, too, studied crash injuries. It was my full time occupation for 9 years in the U.S. Air Force, and then for another year as a member of Wyle Laboratories, under contract to the newly formed National Highway Safety Bureau (now called the National Highway Traffic Safety Administration).

Later, for another 8 years, I dealt with trauma of many origins, first as an emergency physician and then as a director of emergency medical services. Finally, these past 9 years I have actively consulted with both the plaintiff and defense bars in the medical-legal aspects of crash injury causation, studying in detail the mechanical causes and the medical outcomes of at least another several hundred crashes.

All that has happened since and in good part because I read Dr. Kulowski's book about crash injuries.

CHAPTER 0

INTRODUCTION

This chapter will introduce you to what this book is about, what this book is not about, how this book is organized, and how you may want to use it. (Now you understand why I labeled it Chapter Zero. On the other hand, it will probably save you time if you read this chapter first.)

WHAT THIS BOOK IS ABOUT

This book is about crash injuries. Therefore, when we discuss different body regions — the extremities, spine, chest, abdomen and head — we will consider only those injuries that are commonly related to crashes. We will not discuss injuries only because they are common, such as the Colles' fracture of the wrist (probably *the* most common adult fracture), because while it is a common fracture, it is not common in car crashes.

This book is written for anyone with an interest in crash injuries: physician, nurse, engineer, consumer advocate, attorney, insurance claim adjuster, paramedic or whomever: anyone with an interest in what happens in crashes and how the injuries they cause come about. By explaining how crash injuries occur this book may also hold interest for anyone concerned with preventing or minimizing crash injuries.

This book should explain why certain injuries may be expected in specific crash conditions and how specific injuries occur. Of special interest may be the patterns of injuries which may characterize use, non-use, or failure of certain restraint systems. Injury patterns also may help to establish the occupant's location within the vehicle. (Not all drivers will admit to being the driver; not all occupants were located where they say they were located.)

This book, as it claims in one of its titles, is a primer, and it therefore will usually limit itself to first principles and primary concepts. Bold print will be used to indicate that we are dealing with a general rule.

When I was teaching, I believed that if understanding and clarity were in conflict, clarity should prevail. Students need "facts" to hang their hats on, and, in a sense, the reader here is a student. So although some argument will be presented, I will not even try to give all sides of potential or existing arguments and I shall not hesitate to oversimplify a complex concept. My belief in oversimplification in preference to confusion will apply also to figures and tables from referenced sources that I have usually and unhesitatingly oversimplified.

Because I do not like to go to the back of a book to hunt references, I indulge myself by placing each chapter's bibliography at the end of each chapter. I hope that repetition of some references is a small enough price to pay for the convenience of their locations.

Perhaps the greatest consequence of the diversity of persons with a need to know what is going on in crash injuries may be that we all use essentially different and largely unrelated archives. We are not only trained to look at the same events differently, we also publish a lot of data, analyses and conclusions for our peers, and it is improbable that such papers will be readily found and read by non-peers, and if read, that they will be wholly understood by other disciplines as presented and published for peers.

This book then also is my attempt to bridge at least some of the archival and training gaps in the field of crash injury causation.

WHAT THIS BOOK IS NOT ABOUT

This book is not intended as a mathematics, physics, anatomy, engineering, or formal text of any sort. It is, as it said it is, a primer on the why and how crash injuries happen.

This book also is not a compendium, nor are its references exhaustive. I admit to difficulty in determining which references are most important or most useful or most clearly written, and I doubt that I have succeeded in picking well between the best references. It is also true that there are many perfectly awful papers that have been published, but even an awful paper may have an important or useful portion that I must use. Therefore, I have attempted to meet the reference problem head-on: I have used as *few* references as I possibly could. This book is, after all, just a primer.

Anatomy is not taught here, although there must and will be some review of the subject. Anatomy, like physics, is available to you, the reader, in many wonderful texts and, unlike physics, in even more wonderful anatomy atlases. Recommended reference texts and atlases are provided both in the text and in appropriate chapter bibliographies.

There are some sections where considerable anatomic or pathomechanic detail is given and other sections where large anatomic regions are dismissed handily. The reason for such disparities is my belief that the regions here dealt with in detail have been given short shrift as crash injuries and that too little has been done to prevent some easily preventable injuries. Examples of this surely are the many, often severely disabling extremity injuries.

HOW THIS BOOK IS ORGANIZED

The Table of Contents should tell all you would want to know about how this book is organized. But you may also want to know that I think of crash injuries in terms of the *vehicles,* the *victims,* and the *velocities,* and that is how we will look at them. Our crash course on car crash should give you some feel for what happens in the brief and terrible moments of a car crash. We will then have a crash course on principles of trauma, of how we tear and break, of mechanisms of tissue injury. From there it is a short hop to specific injuries and injury mechanisms, for extremities, abdomen, thorax, face/head/brain, and the spine. Finally, we will dip into related topics, such as restraint systems and the concepts of how we measure injury, impairment and disability.

HOW TO USE THIS BOOK

If you have a specific interest, a specific injury, a need to understand a mechanism of injury, by all means skip around and read what you will. But I urge that you first read and understand what happens in a crash, the importance of the crash conditions (direction and magnitude of forces) and how age, sex, restraint systems, location within the vehicle and vehicle size itself — how all of these factors may or may not be causally important to specific injury. In short, I hope that you first read the two early chapters in their entirety before gallivanting through the rest of the book.

CHAPTER 1

A CRASH COURSE ON CAR CRASH

WHAT IS A TYPICAL CRASH?

To understand what happens during a car crash we need to know certain attributes of the car: its weight, speed and direction of travel: and of the crash: how much time did the crash take, which is to say, over what time period did the car's velocity change? We also need to know of the *dynamic passive mechanical characteristics* of what was struck and of what struck it.

Because some cars weigh more than twice as much as others and because their speeds and direction at impact are even more variable than their weights, it would be convenient if we could study a "typical" crash. Perhaps it was the convenience of studying a single, hopefully "typical" car crash that motivated the National Highway Traffic Safety Administration (hereinafter called NHTSA) to select a 30 mile per hour flat frontal barrier collision as its primary test condition. Later, in its New Car Assessment Program (NCAP), NHTSA upped the speed to a 35 mile per hour frontal barrier collision as the method by which NHTSA assesses the crashworthiness of any particular vehicle or compares its crashworthiness to other vehicles, using standard dummies as car occupants and measuring various loads to which the occupant dummies are subjected.

However, there is no "typical crash."

If we use fatal accidents — that is, one or more deaths per accident — then more than half of all fatal accidents involve only one car and at least half of these are not frontal collisions[1]. When two or more cars are involved (some 42 percent of fatal crashes) about 1 crash in 3 is a frontal crash.

When both single and multi-vehicle fatal frontal crashes are combined, we find that the "typical" frontal crash occurs less than half the time; in fact, closer to 40 percent of the time. Pure lateral collisions (3 o'clock and 9 o'clock) account for more than pure frontal collisions by some ten percent[1].

The U.S. Fatal Accident Reporting System which provides the above statistics describes only the vehicles in which the fatality occurred. We will therefore turn to West Germany, where some 12,000 traffic accidents were studied in which either an injury or a death occurred and for which the point of contact was recorded for both cars in the car-to-car accidents[2]. Let me note in passing that in more than half of the injuries and half of the deaths involving cars, the injuries and deaths were not occupants of the cars: they were pedestrians, bicyclists and motorcyclists. The West German study was reported in 1985.

Considering both vehicles — in car-to-car crashes — and the contact point in single car crashes, then 58 percent of car-to-car crashes and 49 percent of single car crashes were frontal collisions. (On the other hand, both types of car crashes together caused less than one-half of all deaths due to cars and less than one-half of all injuries due to cars.)

Of course, not everyone agrees with these statistics or my interpretation of them. As an example, Backaitis et al[3], using yet another data base, the National Crash Severity Study (NCSS) for 1979, calculated that 79 percent of passenger car accidents in that data base involved frontal structures of a car striking another object.

In any event, we will here use the frontal *barrier* crash to study the time sequence of crash events in the following sections because so very many controlled test frontal crashes have been studied and their events reported in great detail (e.g. NCAP). But we will be aware that a frontal barrier crash is a poor representative of all crashes, that it is not necessarily the most common crash, that it may not at all be the best measure of crashworthiness, and that it is more of a convenience than a reality to "typify" car crashes.

THE FRONTAL BARRIER CRASH: THE TIME EPOCH

All of the deformation of metal, all of the tearing and crushing of flesh occurs, quite literally, in the blink of an eye. In about one tenth of a second, to be precise.

In order to study this relatively brief time period we divide it into units of one-thousandths of a second, called "milliseconds." Thus a typical frontal crash begins and is over in about 100 to 120 milliseconds, the duration increasing with increasing vehicle curb weight and with increasing delta v[3]; ("delta v" is further defined below and should be taken to mean an essentially instantaneous change in velocity).

THE FRONTAL BARRIER CRASH: VELOCITY CHANGE ("DELTA V"), ACCELERATION, DECELERATION AND CRUSH

When we say "speed" we mean miles per hour, or feet per second or meters per second and the like. We are dealing only with magnitude, with how much speed there is or was. When we deal only with magnitude, we are dealing with what the physicist calls a "scalar" term, here the attribute of amount of speed.

When we say "velocity" we mean miles per hour (or the like) *in a given direction*. That is, to the attribute of magnitude we have added the attribute of direction, and the physicist calls this a "vector term," with attributes of both amount of speed and the direction of travel. Thus a change in velocity may entail a change in speed or a change in direction of travel or changes in both speed and direction of travel.

The term "delta v" will be used throughout this book to represent an "instantaneous change in velocity." The Greek letter "delta" is a mathematical shorthand term for "change" and "v" is a similar shorthand term for velocity. (Don't be thrown by Greek letters or shorthand; there is no mystery here. An instantaneous change in velocity is either a very sudden increase — as when one is standing still bent over and is booted in the rear — or a very brief decrease in velocity, as in a frontal barrier crash, truly an "instantaneous change in velocity.")

As to the terms "acceleration" and "deceleration," they are the same thing; only the direction is opposite for each. That is, the rate of change of velocity is termed acceleration or deceleration depending on whether it increases velocity (+ acceleration, or "acceleration") or decreases it (- acceleration or "deceleration"). While speed is a scalar quantity and has only the dimensions of distance and time, (e.g., say, miles per hour, or feet per second), and velocity is a vector quantity with dimensions therefore of both speed and direction (e.g., say, miles per hour at 90 degrees, or due east), acceleration has the dimensions of distance per unit of time per unit of time, say miles per hour per second or feet per second per second. Acceleration then is the *rate of change of velocity*.

It is surely intuitively clear that the more violent the crash (the heavier the vehicles, the faster they are traveling, etc.), the more deformation and distortion of metal occurs. An old and very approximate rule-of-thumb for delta v's from about 10 to 50 miles per hour (mph) gives "1.5 mph of delta v for every 1 inch of frontal crush;" thus for a 30 mile per hour delta v collision into a rigid barrier we would expect about two feet of vehicle crush, which is about what we do get[4][5].

As so succinctly stated by the British authors W. Johnson and A.G. Mamalis[6], long, moving, uniform tubular structures colliding end-on with flat, stationary bodies

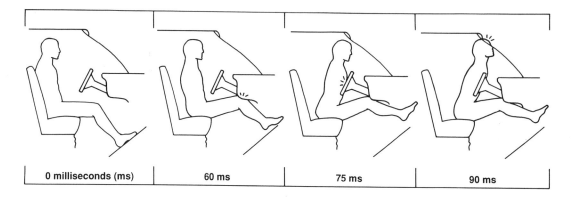

Figure 1A
UNRESTRAINED DRIVER

A car traveling at 30 miles per hour undergoes a frontal crash into an immovable flat barrier. The illustration above depicts the motion of a *dummy* driver as derived from a 2 degree of freedom computer program. Human unrestrained drivers would be expected to have similar but certainly not identical displacement through time.

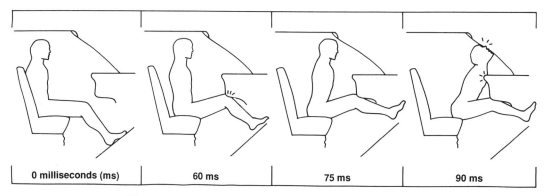

DERIVED IN PART FROM REFERENCES 3 AND 7, CHAPTER 1

Figure 1B
UNRESTRAINED RIGHT FRONT OCCUPANT

As in 1A, this is a computer-derived-but-hand-drawn representation of a *dummy's* motion in the right front seat of a vehicle crashed into an immovable flat barrier.

Pure frontal crashes into an immovable flat barrier are not common events. Dummies have passive dynamic mechanical characteristics that are different from yours and mine. The computer program utilizes an averaged vehicle stiffness and applies it to project movements of a human surrogate in an improbable crash situation. This is, however, as usual and as good a representation of frontal occupants' displacements-through-time in frontal crashes as we are used to dealing with in this field of endeavor.

You should use these representations of a typical frontal crash for what they are: *approximations*, and of dummys' movements at that.

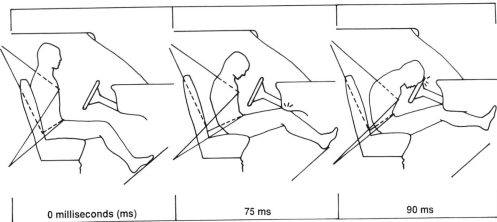

0 milliseconds (ms)   75 ms   90 ms

DERIVED IN PART FROM REFERENCES 3 AND 7, CHAPTER 1

Figure 2
THE RESTRAINED DRIVER

Again, this is a computer derived projection of the movement of a 3 point seat belt restrained dummy driver in a 30 mph frontal flat barrier crash.

Note that the driver moved forward despite the restraints, striking knees and head. If you check crash tests of restrained driver dummies you will find that this is usual and customary. If you check figure 3 you will see why we so often hit parts of the car interior in front of us in frontal crashes; it is because the car was designed without apparent concern for the *flail volume* of the occupant.

What is a flail volume? Why, the text and figures 4, 5 and 6 will deal with that. But what it means is that *we are expected to hit these portions of the car interior, even when we are restrained by the available seat belt system.* We are just expected to hit them somewhat less hard when we are restrained than when we are unrestrained. Note too that there are no requirements to provide padding for these expected contact areas of the car. This may well bother you to find that this is so as much as it bothered me to learn of it.

Now you may look at airbags with a new level of appreciation for the gas filled cushion they may some day provide for you before you put your face into the steering assembly in a frontal crash.

will experience resisting forces which would be inversely proportional to their lengths (if mass, density, cross-sectional area are the same), "then this last expression implies that ships are relatively safe, railway coaches and aircraft less so, and that motor cars are dangerous." Of course it also implies that longer cars are safer than shorter cars, a truism we will find in the next chapter and which I also believe to be intuitively clear.

What seems not to be intuitively clear is that the same crush that occurs to a vehicle in a frontal barrier crash of 30 mph delta v is apportionable, as between say the car and the barrier, (the barrier not being crushed and the car sustaining 2 feet of crush), or between two cars of equal mass, each traveling 30 mph, or between two cars of equal mass, one traveling at 45 mph and the other at 15 mph — in each case above, each car would sustain an equal delta v and equal crush, of about 2 feet. If you do not understand this to be so, you might reread this and reflect upon it until you do understand it, for it is important that you understand that this is so.

THE FRONTAL BARRIER CRASH: WHAT HAPPENS TO THE UNRESTRAINED DRIVER AND RIGHT FRONT SEAT OCCUPANT?

In simple terms, the car slows as its front end is crushed and then the car stops when its kinetic energy ("motion energy") is used up by crush. The unrestrained occupant does not slow and stop, and instead, continues to travel along the same trajectory that it was traversing before the car slowed and stopped, until the occupant in motion hits the stopped or slowing vehicle's interior. It may be said that the car stops before the occupant does; that the occupant effectively "runs into" the slowing or stopped car interior. (The collision of the occupant and the vehicle interior has been termed by some "the second collision." The "first collision" is, of course, that of the vehicle into whatever it strikes.)

Figure 1 shows an unrestrained and figure 2 a restrained fiftieth percentile male dummy (about 5'-8" and about 180 pounds), each in representative drivers' seats set at the mid-position of their travel. The average car, if there is such a thing, has six or seven inches of front-to-rear seat travel on tracks. It is generally set so that the "average" male driver has the seat positioned at mid-position.

The fiftieth percentile male dummy is derived from anthropologic studies of our population. It is a fictional creature for whose measurements it is estimated that half of all adult males are dimensionally larger in all dimensions and half of all adult males are dimensionally smaller in all dimensions.

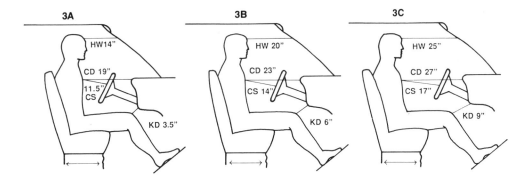

ALL SEATS IN MID POSITION FOR FIFTIETH PERCENTILE MALE DUMMY
RANGE OF DIFFERENCES FOR DISTANCES ATTRIBUTABLE TO
VEHICLE DESIGN DIFFERENCES
DATA DERIVED FROM REFERENCE 7, CHAPTER 1

KEY:
HW = HEAD TO WINDSHIELD
CD = CHEST TO DASHBOARD
CS = CHEST TO STEERING WHEEL
KD = KNEE TO DASHBOARD

Figure 3A, 3B, 3C
DISTANCES TO INTERIOR CONTACTS FOR A DRIVER

This figure shows typical changes in average distances from portions of a driver to portions of a car's interior.

These figures contain no secret information. These measurements can be made by anyone with a measuring tape and a car.

When combined with expected forward motions, which are published in unclassified references such as ref.[11] for example, there is no way to expect that even restrained occupants will not strike these interior structures in front of them in a frontal crash. The only reasonable question, if there is such, may be "How hard will they hit?".

Another reasonable question may be "Why is this so?" After all, we do have the option of moving the windshield, the steering wheel and the dashboard to a distance further from the driver. Why are they so often set where we will surely hit them?

In fact, we know that one may be the fiftieth percentile in height and be the thirtieth percentile in thigh length, or the seventy-fifth percentile in weight, and so forth, which is one reason why I refer to it as a fiction. The other reason that I refer to test percentile dummies as fictions is to emphasize that the anthropomorphic dummies used in car crash tests may look like humans, because their coverings are tinted skin-color and faces are put on with noses and occasionally other features, but in terms of everything from their percentile dimensions to their passive dynamic mechanical characteristics, they are fictions. They are still but inadequate biomechanical surrogates for humans; *they are not human equivalents!* One should either never extrapolate directly from what happened to a dummy in a test to what happens to humans, or do so only with the greatest caution, a caution not always or not even often respected or present in the open literature.

Figure 3 shows the spacing between the dummys' chests and the steering wheel hubs, as well as the distances from the dummys' knees to the dashboards (i.e., instrument panels) and the distances from the dummys' heads to the windshields. These are average distances, so the ranges of these of distances are also given, as derived from vehicles of different sizes, weighing from 2,000 to 5,000 pounds test weight[7], for the smallest occupant volume (figure 3 a), for the average (figure 3 b) and for the largest occupant envelope (figure 3 c).

Figure 1 then shows how these dummies are displaced during the 100 or so thousandths of a second (100 milliseconds) of a 30 mile per hour frontal barrier crash. An unrestrained driver-dummy in succession will strike its knees to the dash, then its chest to the steering wheel and finally, its head into and through the windshield. Note, too, (in figure 2) that the restrained driver-dummy strikes the rim or the hub of the steering wheel with its head or face. Let me emphasize that this head-to-wheel contact by a restrained driver, whether a dummy or you or me, is the rule, rather than the exception, that it occurs well over 95 percent of the time in crash tests in the absence of airbags (see almost any NCAP test).

In a frontal crash, the only question is that of "how hard?", not "whether" the head of a restrained driver will strike the steering wheel. Another question may be, "If it is your head, or your face, would you rather it strike the steering wheel or an airbag?"

The time course of displacement of dummies during frontal crash was derived from many sources, but for the purposes here, largely from a paper by Backaitis, DeLarm and Robbins[3] and partially from another by Mackay[8]. It should be emphasized that the displacements are from a computer model that predicts the time course of a dummy's displacement during crash in only two dimensions (the MVMA-2D program). Let it also be emphasized that the representation here is *an approximation of a computer model that predicts what dummies would do in frontal crashes.* And most recent literature on this same subject does about the same inexact, tenuous thing, which is not necessarily representative of the real world. Again let me state; it is a model that attempts to predict what motions dummies have in two dimensions and does not (cannot) claim that these motions are necessarily the same as that of people moving in three dimensions, in differing precrash positions, and different precrash pretensioning. That we use such modeling at all is because we do not wish to use people in test crashes.

THE FRONTAL BARRIER CRASH: AN UNRESTRAINED DUMMY DRIVER'S KINEMATICS, IN SLOW MOTION

See figure 1. At zero time (0 ms, or 0 milliseconds) the front of the car has just contacted the barrier. By 90 ms the front of the car has been crushed about 2 feet; *which is to say that the car has essentially stopped its forward motion.* During this brief period the occupant-dummy continues its forward travel at 30 miles per hour (about 44 feet per second), its forward motion impeded only slightly by the friction between the dummy's bottom and the seat pan, until it strikes its knees into the dashboard at about 60 milliseconds, causing the lower body to abruptly stop its forward travel and causing the upper torso to flex (bend forward), the upper torso striking the steering assembly at about 75 ms into the crash.

The head and neck flex further when the chest strikes the steering wheel and then contact (often passing into and through) the plane of the windshield, shattering the windshield, and, on occasion, parts of the head and face too, at about 90 milliseconds. Another way to visualize this is to understand that the crash started out with the head 2 feet or so from the windshield, at its ''normal'' driving position. Then, in the crash event, the car stopped after 2 feet of travel and the head after 4 feet of travel. Clear? If not, you ought to re-read and reflect upon this section on slow-motion collision kinematics.

To portray the above scenario a bit more accurately, we should appreciate that we took the vehicle from 30 mph to 0 mph in 2 feet, for an average deceleration of 15 G (i.e., 15 times the ''pull of gravity'' on Earth).

In truth, the collapse of the front of the car was not that linear; rather it collapsed in a non-uniform fashion, the bumper and grille structures collapsing quite easily and the structural members a foot or so further inward being much stiffer. So the actual deceleration would be rather non-linear, with transient decelerations of both lower and higher levels. We also assumed that the 30 mph barrier crash did not deform the passenger compartment at all and that there was no intrusion into this compartment by any structural member in front of the passenger compartment. In many vehicles, however, especially those below say, 2,400 pounds curb weight, I should not be surprised if the toe pan or the floor pan buckled, slapping the soles of the dummy's feet — and, if the feet were human feet — causing grievous foot and ankle fractures. Nor should I be surprised if, especially in small compact and sub-compact cars, the steering assemblies moved rearward in the frontal crash, intruding into the driver's space, or even into the driver. I should not be surprised because I have too often seen just that.

That the occupant struck first the knees, then the chest and lastly, the head, has great consequences. As Mackay has pointed out[8], when the knees struck the dash (at 60 ms), the dash was still travelling forward at about 10 feet per second, while the knees had a velocity of 44 feet per second, yielding a delta v of about 34 feet per second for the knees (with a deceleration of about 70 G and a crush of about 3 inches into the dash). When the chest struck the steering wheel, there was a similar delta v for the chest of about 41 feet per second (28 miles per hour) if, of course, the steering wheel column collapsed about 4 inches, complying with the appropriate Federal Motor Vehicle Safety Standard.

Finally, and perhaps most importantly, since head injury is often said to be the most common injury to vehicle occupants and the most common cause of death for them[9][10], note that the head didn't strike the windshield until the car's 2 feet of crush was completed and the car had stopped moving. *The resultant delta v for the head therefore was the full 44 feet per second* (30 miles per hour) as it struck the stationary windshield, penetrating it or bulging it forward some 5 inches, if it was a usual laminate.

In actual field studies it is not uncommon to see the head strike the area just above the windshield, termed "the header." Should the head in the above example have struck the header, the delta v would be unchanged but the deceleration would be above 700 G, as that area is generally unpadded and the local crush of metal would only be about 0.5 inch.

THE FRONTAL BARRIER CRASH: A RESTRAINED DUMMY DRIVER'S KINEMATICS, IN SLOW MOTION

See figure 2. Here the driver dummy will wear the most available and therefore the most commonly employed restraint system, a so called "three point" system (i.e., three attachment points, one of which is a retractor of the webbing). It is also called a "lap/shoulder belt" or a "lap/torso" seat belt, and there are many variations on this theme that will be dealt with later, in a chapter devoted to restraint systems.

As the crash develops and its front end crush ensues, the vehicle slows and the restrained driver initially doesn't, as with the unrestrained driver. But after only a few inches of occupant travel, the occupant-driver's forward motion puts the driver hard against the lap belt, then the torso webbing.

Meanwhile, the car's deceleration has caused a pendulum driven lock-bar to arrest the spool's rotation, generally within 1 inch of spool rotation. Tightening of the webbing still wound around the spool (about 19" or so) allows an additional webbing spool-out, the total amount of spool-out being quite variable but averaging some 2-1/2"[11], to which may be added the belt slack most humans seem to require, about 4-3/4"[11]. Absent devices intended to reduce spool-out, such as webbing clamps or active webbing retractors, the webbing functionally then has 7" or 8" of slack during impact, for one reason or another. Since the webbing attaches at each side of an occupant, the forward motion that may be attributed to belt slack from all of these causes will be one-half of the total slack, or some 3 to 4 inches of forward motion.

The three-point belt restrained driver, as shown in figure 2, then proceeds to strike the surfaces shown in that figure, the main differences from the unrestrained 5'-8" driver being that we expect (hopefully) little or no contact of knee to dash and little or no contact of the chest to the steering wheel. Instead, because the head itself is not restrained and still has some 19" to 24" of forward (horizontal) travel, the restrained driver's head will almost invariably strike the steering assembly, hub or rim (see the first 150 NCAP tests).

In a study clearly intended to answer the question of how (or even why) three-point belt restrained occupants were injured, Dalmotas[12], of Transport Canada, reported on some 314 fully restrained occupants of passenger cars who sustained "moderate" injuries (to be defined later, when we look at the Abbreviated Injury Scale, as "AIS 2"). He found that, of the *fully restrained drivers in frontal collisions, 40 percent had head/face/neck injuries* (and I think many of us expected that), *over 20 percent had shoulder/chest injuries* (I don't think we all had expected that) and *over 20 percent had lower extremity injuries* (and I don't think we expected that either). But then, among other reasons, perhaps real live drivers weren't all dimensionally of the fiftieth percentile, were they?

Nearly all of the drivers' head/face/neck injuries were from striking the steering assembly.

Half of the chest/abdomen injuries were from striking the steering assembly, the other half were caused by the torso restraint webbing itself — including rib and sternum fractures — while nearly all of the knee injuries (some one-third of all lower extremity injuries) were sustained by knee contact to the dash or steering column, and all of this occurred at crashes within the 30 mph barrier test conditions. We will save discussion of seat belt restraint effectiveness for later chapters about vehicles, their designed occupant flail space, and restraint systems.

THE FRONTAL BARRIER CRASH: THE RIGHT FRONT SEAT PASSENGER, UNRESTRAINED AND RESTRAINED, IN SLOW MOTION

The main difference between the driver and the right front occupant is in the interior spacing, in the absence of the steering assembly. The horizontal distance from the passenger's chest to the dash/instrument panel varies from about 18" to nearly 27," averaging about 21" (see figure 3).

Without the steering assembly to ride down, the unrestrained passenger will, as does the driver, strike knees-to-dash at about 60 milliseconds after the car's front end begins to crush. The resultant impact velocities are about 15 mph for the knees into the dash, about 20 mph for the chest (or upper abdomen) into the dash, and some 28 mph into (and often through) the windshield[3].

The restrained right front occupant of "average" size ought not impact anything, but as Dalmotas has made clear in his article "Mechanisms of Injury to Vehicle Occupants Restrained by Three Point Belts[12]," restrained right front occupants certainly do impact the car interior. For "moderate" injuries, (Abbreviated Injury Scale equal to or greater than AIS 2), he found 39 percent of the injured right front occupants had head, face or neck injuries, 30 percent had chest injuries, 64 percent had abdominal or pelvic injuries and 50 percent had lower extremity injuries, the latter primarily from dashboard contact.

As much as I am attempting to keep this simple, the truth is that all of the above impact estimates are significantly changed by precrash braking, the seated height of the occupant, the location of the seat on its track, seat belt slack, and the quite variable and specific layout of the occupant volume ("flail space," see figure 3).

Yes, we will further discuss the effectiveness and lack of effectiveness of the three point restraint system throughout this book, especially in the section on restraint systems.

But restraint systems can only restrain motion, which is to say that they limit rather than prevent all motion. The amount of space provided for the enevitable movement of occupants at crash will ultimately define one characteristic of crashworthiness, that of "occupant flail space," which will be discussed in the next chapter.

BIBLIOGRAPHY

1. Fatal Accident Reporting System 1989. *NHTSA, DOT HS* 807693, Table 6-10, 1990.
2. Danner, M., Langwieder, K. and W. Schmelzing: Aspects in optimizing car structures and passenger protection by a comprehensive analysis of car-to-car and car-to-object collisions. *SAE* paper 850514, 1985.
3. Backaitis, S.H., DeLarm, L. and D.H. Robbins: Occupant kinematics in motor vehicle crashes. *SAE* paper 820247, 1982.
4. Campbell, K.L.: Energy basis for collision severity. *SAE* paper 740565, 1974.
5. Prasad, A.K.: Energy dissipated in vehicle crush — a study in using the repeated test technique. *SAE* paper 900412, 1990.
6. Johnson, W. and A.G. Mamalis: *Crashworthiness of vehicles.* Mechanical Engineering Publications Ltd. London, p. 14, 1978.
7. Cohen, D.S., Jettner, E. and W.E. Smith: Light Vehicle Frontal Impact Protection. *SAE* paper 820243, 1982.
8. Mackay, M., in: Biomechanics of impact trauma. *AAAM & IRCOBI* June 4-6, 1984.
9. Malliaris, A.C., Hitchcock, R. and J. Hedlund: A search for priorities in crash protection. *SAE* paper 820242, 1982.
10. Scott, W.E.: Epidemiology of head and neck trauma in victims of motor vehicle accidents, in *Head and Neck Injury Criteria*, Washington, D.C., March 26-27, 1981.
11. Mitzkus, J.E. and H. Eyrainer: Three point belt improvements for increased occupant protection. *SAE* paper 840395, 1984.
12. Dalmotas, D.J.: Mechanisms of injury to vehicle occupants restrained by three point belts. *SAE* paper 801311, 1980.

CHAPTER 2

VEHICLES, VICTIMS AND VELOCITIES

THE VEHICLE: GENERAL COMMENTS AND CONCEPTS

No one, I believe, deliberately starts out to build a vehicle that is not crashworthy.

It is probably also true that not everyone who builds automotive vehicles starts out with the intention of building the most crashworthy car that it is possible or even practicable for them to build.

In fact, we know that, for 1984-88 cars, the death rate between different models varied by as much as 800 or 900 percent[1]. As between the Chevrolet Corvette Coupe and the Volvo 240 Station Wagon, for example, *an occupant involved in an accident was 9 times more likely to die in the Chevrolet Corvette than in the Volvo station wagon*. The curb weights of these two vehicles are almost the same, within a hundred pounds of each other. The 9 times difference in car occupant crash survival may be termed "crashworthiness." The 1984-88 Volvo station wagon clearly had a lot more of this attribute than did the contemporary Chevrolet Corvette Coupe.

Well, that doesn't seem fair, comparing a station wagon with a sports car. Okay. We'll compare a couple of small cars with each other. How about a Saab 900, with a Chevrolet Sprint (both 1984 to 1988 four door models, classified as "small cars")? The Chevrolet Sprint had 9 times the death rate of the Saab 900 per 10,000 cars registered[1].

Why should this be so? Is it possible that other priorities may precede concern for life and limb? Who oversees priorities?

To understand why cars can vary so in their crashworthiness, we need start with some philosophical distinctions, improbable as that may seem for a discussion of automotive vehicles. But cars and trucks and the like are made and marketed by very large corporations. Very large corporations are very large institutions, controlling large numbers of people, great physical and monetary assets, and, on occasion, governments. And all large institutions have their own orthodoxies, often different from other large institutions, such as governments.

For example, a very, very large corporation — the original AT&T in about the year

1965 — had assets, people and cash flow that made it equivalent to the 13th state of the Union, and certainly larger than many of the countries of South America[2]. It was, in fact, a very large *government*, controlling a large number of people, and a large amount of assets.

Automobile manufacturers are not quite that large, but they are still huge, potent institutions. And they have good people who do believe (must believe!) as Charles Wilson, then president of General Motors, surely did believe, when, in testifying before the Senate committee that confirmed him as Secretary of Defense under Eisenhower, said "for years I thought what was good for our country was good for General Motors, and vice versa. The difference did not exist."

I am attempting to make clear that what may be good for sales may be bad for occupant safety. When style and safety clash, safety is a doubtful victor.

Perhaps too, this is reflected in the very substance of the National Highway Traffic Safety Administration (NHTSA), created by our government to reduce our nation's mind-numbing long record of vehicular carnage by establishing *minimum* automotive safety criteria. NHTSA was effectively gutted even as it was born, the Act making the Administrator of the National Highway Traffic Safety Administration, the organization's chief operating manager, a political appointee.

In its history since its creation in 1966 (the National Traffic and Motor Vehicle Safety Act of 1966 and the Highway Safety Act of 1966; 80 Stat. 718 and 731), to my knowledge and belief only the first Administrator, Dr. William Haddon, Jr., knew the first thing about motor safety, or had any experience, training or even interest in the subject. Since then there have been a variety of journalists, bureaucrats, businessmen, ex-military officers and the like, generally qualified neither by experience nor training in the field of automotive safety. Perhaps my years in emergency rooms, dealing with wrecked bodies and wrecked lives caused by uncrashworthy wrecked cars, make the appointment of NHTSA administrators qualified only by their ownership of political debt a level of political cynicism beyond my understanding.

The above was written not as some form of therapeutic-ventilation for me, (although I do think it helped!), but rather because we must understand these events and concepts before we can begin to understand why there exists at all some of the vehicle features and characteristics that we will now discuss.

The maldesign of a motor vehicle is not in and of itself proof that an evil intent was its cause, even when maldesign causes, as often it does, unnecessary deaths and injuries. Maldesign may occur because insufficient engineering hours were spent on occupant safety, or safety considerations were given no clout when conflicting with style or cost of fabrication; there are many reasons that may be supposed without creating an active intent to do harm. But explain these reasons, if you will, not to me, but to those who are dead or disabled, without good cause.

THE VEHICLE: CRASHWORTHINESS

We will look at cars and the concept of crashworthiness from the viewpoints of:

1) Crash Energy Management,
2) Car Size,
3) Occupant Volume ("Flail Space"), and
4) Human Factors.

Crash Energy Management

Crash energy is "kinetic energy," literally the energy of the cars due to their motion (from the Greek "kinetikos"). This motion-derived energy is equal to one-half the product of a car's mass (as "pounds") times the square of its velocity ("as feet per second"), so kinetic energy may be expressed in units of foot-pounds. This energy is also expressed more graphically in the amount of vehicle crush that occurs in any accident. It may be said that **the amount of car crush is a direct expression of crash energy**. And it may also be said that by crash energy management we therefore also mean car crush management.

To the extent that we can surround the passenger compartment with crushable material, stuff whose rate of deformation is both helpful and predictable, to that extent we can provide delta v's that are survivable, or even low enough to prevent injury.

By simple inspection of any car we can see that there's a fair amount of space for crush to occur in the front and in the back, but not very much space at all on the sides of a car. That observation alone may explain why, in the 1989 Fatal Accident Reporting System (the last FARS available at this writing), more than 40 percent of multi-vehicle fatalities were side collisions to the struck car[3].

The engineering of the stiffness, amount, shape and location of what will be struck and crushed in accidents may be termed "crash energy management." This engineering determines (and predicts!) the force environment to which crashed vehicle's occupants will be subjected. It also determines (and again predicts!) where and how much intrusion may be expected in the occupant's space. Clearly, poor crash energy management in the design of a vehicle may cause otherwise preventable deaths. There are, however, great engineering subtleties in this design area, far beyond the scope of either this treatise or my own knowledge, and an appropriate level of automotive engineering skill should be consulted for such analysis.

Less subtle, however, is what the automotive trade euphemistically terms "downsizing," i.e., making cars smaller. Clearly, the size of a vehicle relates to its crashworthiness, so we shall look at the implications of car size in the next section.

But let me again remind you that all of the elements that make a car crashworthy, from size, through controlled stiffness, through interior padding, all are at the option and pleasure of the car manufacturer. To claim, as I've heard claimed, that a grossly uncrashworthy vehicle "met all (minimum) Federal Safety Standards" is simple denial that the manufacturer has any social conscience of his own, or has any obligation for decency beyond the minimum demanded by law. In fact, we daily prove with spilled blood that grossly uncrashworthy vehicles can be built that comply well with existing Federal Motor Vehicle Safety Standards.

Car Size

When grandpa said "I like large cars because they are safer than small cars" he was absolutely right; large cars are safer than small cars[4].

Car manufacturers have been under considerable Federal pressure to increase the gas mileage of the "average" car produced in a given year. They have met this demand partly by making the cars more efficient and partly by making new cars lighter in weight for a given wheelbase, but largely by making the average fleet vehicle smaller[5].

Simply put, the smaller the car, the less space available for crush to occur before some portion of the car intrudes into the occupant volume. When metal and flesh then compete to occupy the same space, the flesh always loses; injury or death is the penalty paid. Is this simplistic explanation true? Probably.

Jones and Whitfield showed that a seat belted driver gains a 25 percent reduction in injury odds for every additional thousand pounds of car weight he drives, while the unrestrained driver gains a 34 percent injury reduction for every additional thousand pounds of car driven[4]. They also state that "the use of restraints in a very small car cannot overcome the weight disadvantage."

Using fatalities only, Leonard Evans of General Motors Research Laboratories studied both two car crashes and "non-two car crashes," comparing the likelihood

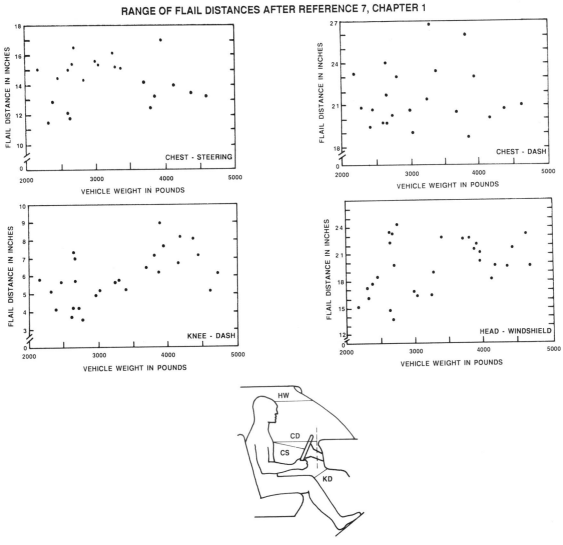

Figure 4
**FRONTAL CRASH INTERIOR CONTACT DISTANCES AND THEIR RELATIONSHIP
TO VEHICLE SIZE**

A look at this figure should make clear that chest-to-steering assembly and chest-to-dash distances bear no relationship at all to vehicle size. Knee-to-dash and head-to-windshield distances fare only a little better: they have *almost* no relationship to size.

I was recently in an older model Honda Prelude that had a good deal more chest-to-steering assembly distance than I have in my older model Lincoln Continental when both driver's seats are in the full-back position. The same was true for knees-to-dash and head-to-windshield distances.

This figure should make it clear to you that a larger, "roomier" and heavier car does not necessarily (or even usually!) provide more volume or more distance for restrained occupant flailing during crash.

of fatality if the involved cars weighed 900 kg (1,980 lbs) or 1,800 kg (3,960 lbs). He found that in "non-two car crashes" the driver was nearly twice as liable (1.7 times as likely) to die in the smaller car; in two car crashes the driver was 4 times as likely to die in the smaller car[6].

In a study from NHTSA in 1987 that used both fatality and injury data bases, different sizes of cars, pickup trucks and vans were compared[7]. It was found that small cars, small pickups and multi-purpose vehicles ("utility" vehicles) had the highest overall injury and involvement rates, while small and standard vans had the lowest. In two vehicle crashes, small cars fared worse and standard vans fared best. *In crashes in all directions, frontal, side and rear, small cars had the highest injury and death rates.*

The most recent statistical work up on this subject that I have found, also done by NHTSA, again showed an increase in fatalities about 4 times greater in "minicompact" cars as compared to "fullsize cars," which themselves showed a substantial fatality increase when compared to "large cars[8]."

Grandpa was right.

Occupant Volume (Flail Space)

About thirty years ago John J. Swearingen, at the Civil Aeronautics Research Laboratories near Oklahoma City, wondered what volume would be defined, what space would be passed through (briefly occupied) by a seated, lap belted occupant who moved his unrestrained upper torso through every possible direction and position that he could reach, i.e., his upper torso was flailed through this volume, as would lap belted crash victims as they flailed about during crashes. His concern was aircraft crashes, but the concept was good for any crash. The studies were published some ten years later[9]. The term "strike envelope" has been applied to this flailed volume, although I prefer and we here use the term "flail volume."

By excluding the upper limbs, such a volume is limited to a radius equal to the occupant's seated height, about 33" for the shortest 1 percentile, about 36" for the 50th percentile, and about 39" for the 99th percentile male[10]. Please understand that when we exclude the upper limbs, we are saying that since we cannot (do not) restrain them, the upper limbs will flail about, striking portions of the car or other occupants, and this may cause injury. But if we include the upper limbs, the occupant volume becomes an irregular hemi-ellipsoid more than 12 feet wide, 6 feet high and 6 feet deep, a flail space so large that we could not even fit it into a car! So, for the moment at least and perhaps into the forseeable future, we don't do anything significant

TWO DIMENSIONAL FLAIL SPACE
FOR LAP BELT RESTRAINED
FIFTIETH PERCENTILE DUMMY

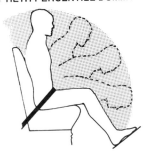

Figure 5
SCALED FROM A 50TH PERCENTILE DUMMY, THIS FIGURE REPRESENTS
HOW THE *UPPER TRUNK* FLAIL IS REPRESENTED IN
TWO DIMENSIONS

This simply shows how the seated, lap belt restrained, upper trunk may be flailed through all forward motions possible in a two-dimensional plane. In the next figure (figure 6) we will show the same manikin placed in the *average forward flail space* available to a front seat occupant.

This illustration is intended to produce *a slice* (a "planar" or 2 dimensional representation) of the volume that could be created if the manikin were to move its unrestrained upper trunk through all motions possible while seated. Because we cannot here show both the forward and backward motions while simultaneously showing side-to-side motion, we chose to show the forward motion only, as a portion of a plane rather than as a portion of a volume.

TWO DIMENSIONAL FLAIL SPACE FOR LAP BELT RESTRAINED
DRIVER AND FRONT SEAT OCCUPANT

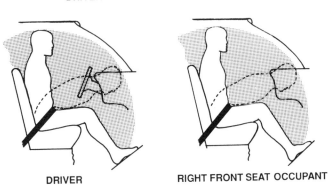

DRIVER   RIGHT FRONT SEAT OCCUPANT

Figure 6
FORWARD FLAIL OF AN "AVERAGE" LAP BELTED FRONT SEAT OCCUPANT
IN A VEHICLE WITH "AVERAGE" SPACE FOR OCCUPANT FLAIL

If nothing else, this illustration shows why we attempt to restrain the upper trunk, which is to say that this shows the impact consequence of wearing only lap belts.

It is intended, however, to show the same lap belt flail volume slice that was introduced to you in figure 5, as it would now apply to either the driver or right front occupant in a frontal collision.

to prevent either upper or lower limb injury.

Perversely, even though we are certain that our arms, legs (and head too!) will flail about during crash, striking various parts of cars' interiors, *we only require vehicle padding for less than 2 percent of the car's interior!*[11]

Figures 3 and 4 show a dangerous, puzzling, and near random relationship between the distances an occupant has to traverse before striking some portion of the interior front of the car and the very size of the car.

It is dangerous because we expect a larger car to have larger space in all directions, but we find that is not necessarily so, that some very small cars provide greater useful interior volume for forward flail than do some cars nearly twice their weight! And the less flail space, the greater the danger.

It is puzzling, because I cannot think of any good reason why this is so.

The near randomness between car size and interior frontal flail space (figure 4) is both apparent and reprehensible. After all, it is reasonably well known that the pedals-to-seat distance is the major determining factor as to where we choose our seat position, that the steering wheel-to-pedal distance influences us far less and that the header proximity matters even less than the steering wheel location[12]. In short, we position our seats for the most comfortable leg position, the seat-to-pedal distance, and we have a fair option to move the steering assembly *as far from the driver as is possible*. Clearly, by using this option we would reduce injuries and save lives; just as clearly, we are not often fully utilizing this important option.

Figure 5 shows a 2 dimensional representation of head and trunk flail space for a lap belt restrained 50th percentile occupant, as in the study done by Swearingen[9]. Figure 6 shows this occupant (flail space) volume when placed into the driver's and the right front occupant's *average* space provided in current vehicles.

We have already seen what a three-point belt restrained driver and right front seat occupant will hit in a frontal crash, each moving in a largely predictable trajectory (see figures 1 and 2, chapter one). More importantly, we have just now found that **there is little or no relationship between vehicle size and the flail space allowed the front seat occupants** (figures 3a, 3b, 3c and 4). This lack of relationship between a vehicle's size and its roominess for occupants, at least with regard to frontal crash, is both unexpected and unexplainable.

Why should a 3,600 pound, so called "full-size" car, have *less* space before the driver's head hits the steering wheel than a Nissan Sentra that weighs barely 2,200 pounds, or a Honda Civic, also at 2,200 pounds curb weight? And the same is true for knee-to-dash, or chest-to-dash space (see also[13]).

To me, the implications of this disparity between the size of a vehicle and the interior room permitted a restrained occupant to flail are very great indeed. Because we know that fully restrained occupants in frontal crashes more often than not strike the steering assemblies, dash, or A pillars (the posts on each side of the windshield), great effort has been expended to eliminate or reduce belt webbing slack, by webbing clamps instead of spool clamps, by pyro-technical retraction of webbing on impact and other means; even inflatable webbing has been tried. The intent should always be to provide space for additional flail before an occupant strikes the vehicle's interior, in order to reduce both the frequency and the level of occupant injuries and deaths[14] [15].

Please go back and study figures 3a, 3b, 3c and 4 if this is not yet apparent to you. But the potential increase in flail space implicit in a longer wheelbase vehicle often is not there, not in the chest-to-dash, not in the head-to-steering wheel, not in the knee-to-dash spaces. Why not? Isn't anyone accountable for flail volumes?

In 1969 there was published a study that used U.S. Air Force volunteer subjects restrained by lap belt and three-point restraints on the "Daisy Decelerator" at Holloman Air Force Base. Sponsored by the relatively new National Highway Safety Bureau, the tests were overseen and reported by members of the National Bureau of Standards (!) as a Society of Automotive Engineers paper[16]. These tests necessarily were kept down to lower level decelerations, although they did go as high as 20 feet per second velocity and 15 G decelerations. General Motors kindly provided photometric analyses of the subjects' displacements through time.

This was a landmark study. It was and still is almost unique in its use of human volunteers and in defining restrained human flail. It should have made clear to the automotive world, the world that reads SAE publications, that *fully restrained occupants have one to two feet of forward head motion as well as substantial forward displacement of chest and hips during even modest frontal crash.* And I think that all of us are anatomically savvy enough to realize that when the hips move forward, so does the thigh bone and the knee bone that connects to it. In short, no one in the automotive world should consider such displacement to be news in the 1990s. Or even the 1980s, or the 1970s.

Let me emphasize that this USAF/NBS study is remarkable in its use of human beings as test subjects, and unique in comparing lap belt vs. lap/torso restraints in terms of the displacements they permit. Additionally, this study used subjects both larger and smaller than the 5'-8" dummy of our standard tests, comparing all of these subjects with two different test dummies. It showed both the great disparity of displacement responses between restrained human subjects of different sizes and between humans and dummies and between different models of dummies. It surely is one of the most important, most useful and most ignored classical reports about restrained human flail response to impact that I have ever read, and I believe that I've surely read almost all of them.

The terms weight and size of vehicle have been used casually and interchangeably because car weight generally is proportional to length (wheelbase), but it would be more accurate to distinguish weight from size. To a large measure, weight is an aggressive car attribute in multivehicle crashes, especially to occupants of other vehicles. Car size, as measured by length, has the potential to protect occupants *if the additional length is used wisely by adding to flail distance by increasing the occupants' flail space.*

Even so, we continue to produce cars of all weights and wheelbases that *we know* have vehicle components, steering wheels, instrument panels, windshields, headers, etc. that are obviously in the pathway of, and are bound to be struck by, head, chest or limbs, even in modest frontal collisions, even for fully restrained occupants. And we apparently do so with the full, if not cheerful, concurrence of the governmental agency that oversees automotive safety.

Perhaps we will understand why this is so when we later review the measures employed by our governing agency to evaluate safety and crashworthiness, one measure being digital (i.e., alive or dead), the other being analog, (the Abbreviated Injury Scale, a measure of threat-to-life, rather than of disability). We will find how the NHTSA measures its success, how their measures may well color the very concept of safety, since a crash victim may be a permanent burden to society, a crippled, mindless shell, all as a result of an auto accident, and yet be scored as a statistical success in the governmental game of vehicular safety measurement.

Human Factors

This term is meant to include everything from reaction time (e.g., how long does it take for us to begin to press the brake pedal after we perceive the need to stop the car?) to the requirements of a seated operator (reach, pedal pressures, etc.). In short, the gamut: from anthropometry, to visual and auditory limits, through the many portions of operating machinery that have, over the course of the last fifty or more years, become the province primarily of general and industrial psychologists, of human factors experts.

Human factors is a necessary consideration in the evaluation of a vehicle's crashworthiness. For example, if an abrupt stop requires brake pedal pressures higher than an elderly, five foot tall woman driver can readily provide, her emergency braking distance may be unreasonably large, may itself be the cause of a crash. Of course the same is true of many factors: visual, auditory, anthropometric, geriatric and more.

This treatise however concentrates on crash *injury* causes, while human factors concentrates on crash causes.

Human factors is concerned with human performance, but because our need in this treatise is to concentrate on the *passive mechanical characteristics* of vehicles and victims, we will not say anything about this important area beyond defining it's territory.

SUMMARY: THE VEHICLE

In our consideration of crash as the vehicle, the victim and the velocity, we have looked at *the vehicle* in terms of its crash energy management (design), its size, its occupant or flail space, and whether consideration was given for human factors in its design. We have noted that crashworthiness must be a governing factor in design; crash energy management simply cannot be retro-fitted as some sort of after-thought. That is, vehicle crush characteristics generally can be modified, but not created, by retrofit.

As to vehicle size, we probably found what we suspected we would find, that death and injury were inversely related to car length or car weight: the smaller the vehicle, the larger its injury and death rate.

We also noted that the occupant volume available for occupant movement and flail during a crash is largely independent of vehicle size (!), a victim's head in a large car quite possibly being closer to say, the windshield, than in a compact car. (The reason for this being so eludes me, but the importance of this fact does not.)

Finally, we only touched on the discipline of Human Factors, concerned with how information is presented to the vehicle operator, how the operator is positioned with regard to controls, and how the operator is burdened by control characteristics.

We will now move on to the victims and how their various characteristics may alter their injury potential.

THE VICTIM: AGE, SEX AND HABITUS

Is there a difference in the incidence of crash injury and death as a function of age?

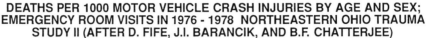

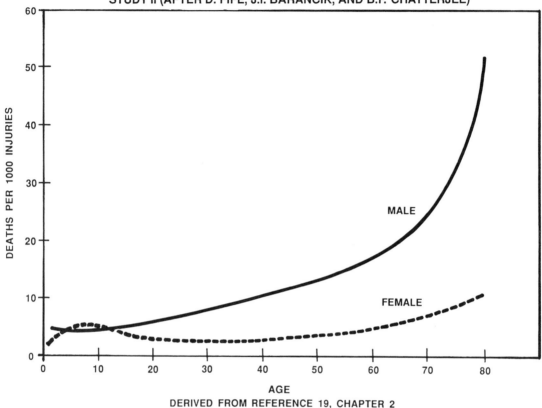

DEATHS PER 1000 MOTOR VEHICLE CRASH INJURIES BY AGE AND SEX; EMERGENCY ROOM VISITS IN 1976 - 1978 NORTHEASTERN OHIO TRAUMA STUDY II (AFTER D. FIFE, J.I. BARANCIK, AND B.F. CHATTERJEE)

DERIVED FROM REFERENCE 19, CHAPTER 2

Figure 7
DEATHS PER 1,000 CRASH INJURIES, BY AGE AND SEX

This is a simplified version of a published graph (ref. 19, chapter 2), which means that I "rounded it off" a bit to make it clearer, at least to me.

It shows that the death rate per 1,000 emergency-room-treated-injuries sustained by males doubles from age 20 to age 40. Then it doubles again from age 40 to age 65, so that a 65 year old male is 8 times more liable to die from a given injury than is a 20 year old male. (This is important news for me since I am a 65 year old male.)

But the death rate per 1,000 ER-treated-injuries doesn't seem to change at all for women as they go from age 20 to 40, and then it begins to rise only a little bit by age 60. By about age 60 to 65, a woman has approximately the same death rate per injury as does the 20 year old male.

Looking at the graph one could make a case that a women's increased death rate from crash injuries doesn't apparently change from puberty until menopause, after which it begins to climb, but far less exponentially than does the male death rate.

By age 80, males have about 50 deaths per 1,000 ER-treated-crash-injuries and females have only one-fifth as many deaths as the males.

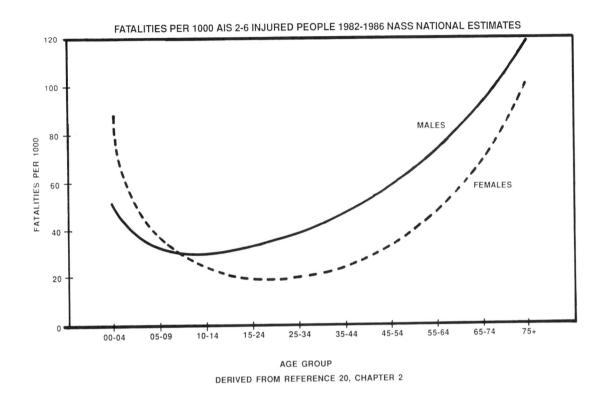

FATALITIES PER 1000 AIS 2-6 INJURED PEOPLE 1982-1986 NASS NATIONAL ESTIMATES

AGE GROUP

DERIVED FROM REFERENCE 20, CHAPTER 2

Figure 8
INJURIES PER 1,000 AIS 2-6 INJURIES ("MODERATE" TO "MAXIMUM"
INJURIES) WITH INCREASING AGE GROUPINGS

Using a quite different injury scale, this graph again illustrates (as did figure 7) that, for AIS injuries of a great range, as derived from NHTSA's National Accident Severity Study, male death rates from crash injuries about doubles between ages 20 and 55 and about doubles again over the subsequent 20 years.

And again, as did figure 7, it shows that from puberty into the AARP years (say, from age 50 onward) females have lower death rates per comparable (?) injury. More interestingly, from puberty to menopause a woman's probability of dying from a given crash injury appears to stay low and only is only slightly changed during the child-bearing ages.

If all of this is true, it raises more questions than it answers. For one thing, it *suggests* that whatever it is that keeps women looking womenly and able to produce babies, (say, female hormones?), are protective during these years, at least with regard to surviving crash injuries, as compared to what keeps men looking manly (say, male hormones?). It also could *suggest*, in alternative, that the same results would obtain if women were more liable to die immediately of injuries that men survived for a while.

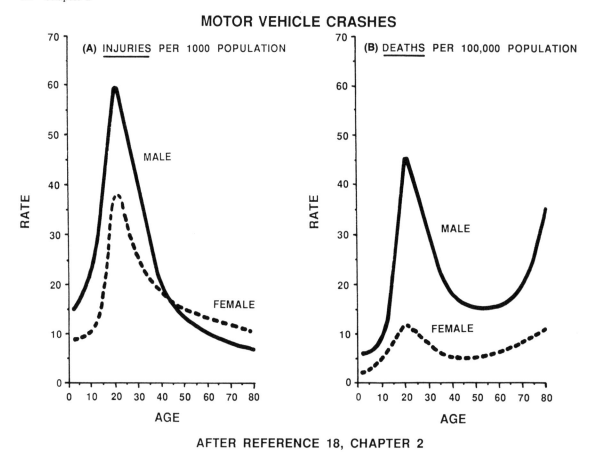

MOTOR VEHICLE CRASHES

AFTER REFERENCE 18, CHAPTER 2

Figure 9
(A&B) MOTOR VEHICLE CRASH INJURIES AND DEATHS
BY SEX AND WITH INCREASING AGE

Why do more men die from crashes than do women? For one thing, from ages 20 to 40, men have twice the crash injury rate (9A), which suggests that they are more often involved in crashes than are women.

Whether that simply means that men drive more miles than women do and are therefore more liable to be involved in an accident or whether it means that men are simply worse drivers than women and therefore are more liable to be involved in an accident or whether men are more liable to be intoxicated while driving than are women or whatever, I cannot say. (I'm not sure that I would dare to say even if I did know.)

Figure 9B shows male dominance in terms of males dominating the motor vehicle death rates from infancy through senescence.

Of particular interest is the finding that the female crash injury rate exceeds that of males from age 40 onward (9A) but the male death rate continues to exceed that of the women even after age 40 (9B), when women sustain more crash injuries than do men.

Does the same injury that we would have survived at age 20 often prove to be lethal at age 40? Do men die of injuries that women the same age will survive? Do women die more often than men in the accident itself? Are we more liable to be injured or die at certain ages more than other ages? Does the same injury have different disability implications as we grow older?

With some variation in confidence when answering each question above, the answer to all of these questions is YES.

Age

Of the various major causes of death in these United States — cardiovascular disease, cancer, motor vehicle injuries, suicide, homicide, and such — the earliest (median) age of death is from motor vehicle injury, at 27 years of age. Only homicide is even close to that, with a 31 year median age[17]. From the late teens to the early twenties, (ages 16-22), two of every five deaths are motor vehicle crash deaths[18].

Death rates from motor vehicles vary widely for different age groups, peaking at three or four times the early years by the late teens and low twenties, for both sexes. Death and injury rates from motor vehicle crash are shown in figures 7 and 8, which are graphically "rounded out" simplifications of graphs from sources[19] and [20].

They indicate a male death rate two to four times that of women by age 30, and the original publication[19] cites a crash injury rate one and one-half times greater for men than women at that same age. Male deaths remain higher than female for all ages, then peak again at ages 65 to 80 years for both sexes.

This disparity in death rates per crash injury raises the question of whether males get involved in more accidents than females, or just worse accidents, or both possibilities. It also raises questions such as "do males or females die most easily (of the same or equivalent injury)?" It would appear that we must consider sex as well as age as major factors, and we do just that in table 1[21].

Sex (and Age, continued)

"In the Netherlands" explains the author of reference[21], "all hospitals join a national registration system of relevant data of each hospitalized casualty based on the WHO-ICD (i.e., World Health Organization, International Classification of Diseases) system." Thus it is our good fortune that in Holland at least, all vehicular accident injuries are classified, recorded, retrievable and available for accident and injury analyses.

Table 1 shows male/female lethality difference, as well as a progressive increase in lethality from ages 25 through about 75. It is in essential agreement with figures 8 and 9. To this we will add table 2, which shows that as we grow older, we spend more time in convalescence for a given injury (and/or, we average more serious injuries for a given accident, as is also suggested by our increasing death rates seen in figures 8 and 9).

Table 1

NUMBER OF FATALITIES PER 100 VICTIMS FOR DIFFERENT AGE GROUPS AND SEXES, 1987 ACCIDENT DATA

	Elderly Crash Victims			Comparison Group
AGE	55-64	65-74	75+	25-44
MALE	16	19	22	11
FEMALE	10	10	14	7

Table 2

LENGTH OF STAY IN HOSPITAL BY AGE AND SEX; 1987 DUTCH HOSPITAL DATA [21], CHAPTER 2

Length Of Stay	Elderly Crash Victims Male	Female	Comparison Group Male	Female
	55+ Years		25-44 Years	
1 Day	3	2	5	4
2-9 Days	32	26	58	53
10-19 Days	29	30	21	27
20-29 Days	16	19	6	7
30 Days Or More	20	23	10	9
	100%	100%	100%	100%
	(N-1724)	(N-1992)	(N-2174)	(N-1065)

From even before puberty and on well afterward, suggests figure 9, men simply get involved and injured in motor vehicle crashes more often than women — at least until age 40 or so — the difference for injuries not being as profound as those for deaths. Is this difference real or a statistical anomaly unique to this northeastern Ohio study[19]?

In early 1988 I wrote to Susan C. Partyka, a fine statistician at NHTSA, about this piquing question. Sometime later, using the National Accident Sampling System (NASS) data base from 1982 to 1986, she sent her findings — "that males have higher injury rates at any particular age, as compared to females," and that the differences are largely accounted for by differences in the severity of the injuries received by each sex[20].

Later that same year, at the 12th International Technical Conference on Experimental Safety Vehicles, in Goteborg, Sweden, L.T.B. van Kampen, using Dutch national accident data banks, reported the age/sex relationship that he found[21]; (see table 1), which is remarkably similar to what we've just discussed above[19] [20].

Finally, (although I believe that we may not yet have final answers), an interesting study[22] by Leonard Evans of General Motors, using the Fatal Accident Reporting System data base and a neat method which he has developed and termed "double-pair comparison," established that *fatality* risk in the age groups from 15 to 45 years is about 25 percent greater for women than for men.

Three studies[19] [20] [21] appear to have shown that males have higher injury rates than women and more deaths per injury, at all ages above 20 years; a fourth[22] has shown that women have higher death rates per accident. The apparent conflict is reconciled if, for whatever reasons, a woman is more liable to die at the time of the accident than is a man, but a man is both more liable to be in an accident and more likely to die of a given, initially survived accident, than is a woman.

But questions unanswered remain: does the woman die more often in an accident than does a man[22] because she is, on the average, physically smaller with, on the average, more easily broken bones, more easily torn soft tissue? Or does the average woman driver have to sit closer to the steering wheel (and therefore the dash and windshield too) in order to reach the accelerator and brake? Or is the woman more often the right front seat occupant than is the man, an inherently more dangerous location? (But the right front seat is *not* an inherently more dangerous seat than that of the driver, according to Malliaris et al[23].) And so forth. What is the data trying to tell us?

Habitus

By habitus we mean both the appearance of a person and the meaning of the appearance. For example, a sick person generally looks sick. And sickly people look as if they are more liable to become sick than people without the poorly defined attributes we refer to as "sickly," i.e., scrawny? poor color? dark rings under the eyes? Whatever it is that somehow suggests to us that someone is "sickly." Conversely, a big strapping lumberjack brimming with all of the color of living in the great outdoors appears not only to be healthy, but strong. We intuitively expect his bones and other tissues to be stronger than one who appears to be less healthy, less strong. Is this really true? If we compared the breaking strengths of a mesomorphic male athlete with an aged osteoporotic female, would her sickly appearing bones break more easily than his, her tissues to tear more easily? Well, generally we would be correct; as we will see shortly, young tissues generally are stronger than aged tissues and people who appear to be strong generally have strong tissues, strong bones, ligaments, tendons, muscles.

Habitus here too includes the person's prior and current medical history, at least to the extent that the history could affect their injury probability and their ability to survive injury. Here injury probability would include everything from age, sex and nutritional history as well as the more obvious chronic diseases, from diabetes to neuromuscular and collagen diseases, all of which would also have profound effects on an injured person's ability to survive an injury or group of injuries.

Selecting as an example bone and ligament strength of the structural spine (vertebrae and intervertebral discs), Nachemson, studying the mechanical properties of isolated human lumbar spine segments, found that age and sex often were overshadowed as factors when compared to the variation within any one age group of the same sex, at least with regard to segment motions and intradiscal pressures resulting from the application of different flexion, extension, bending and torsional moments[24]. However, when the endpoint of such tests went on to breaking these elements, then a clear relationship between age and breaking strength was seen: the older the subject, the lower the breaking strength of both vertebrae and intervertebral discs[25].

What I am saying here is that with regard to passive mechanical characteristics of elastic tissues and bone, the variation from person to person appears to exceed the variation that we could ascribe to age or sex. That is so until we reach breaking strengths, which indeed verify our clinical impressions and experience, in that the older we are, the more readily we break and tear.

Habitus also includes the size of the victim as part of appearance, and this is a bit bothersome. It would be very much more convenient if we were all about the same size.

But we are not all about the same size, and this has made for some awful problems.

One awful problem, for which the NHTSA has provided equally awful solutions, is our variation in height. NHTSA requires only that seats, seat belt restraints, pedal and other controls be based on the 5th to the 95th percentile of adult men and women.

Since the 5th percentile woman is shorter than the 5th percentile man, and the 95th percentile man is taller than the 95th percentile woman, then at least 10 percent of the adult population may not be fitted by seats, seatbelts and reach to controls. If we estimate that the size-excluded adult group is only 5 percent of the 1990 adult population, then according to U.S. Census Bureau estimates, we have excluded or given up on even attempting to fit, about twelve million adults.

Have you ever seen a notice in any car to the effect "NOTICE: THIS VEHICLE IS INTENDED ONLY FOR PEOPLE FROM 4'-11" TO 6'-1". PERSONS NOT WITHIN THESE DIMENSIONS DRIVE OR OCCUPY THESE SEATS AT THEIR OWN RISK?"

Even more significantly, by not fitting well any of the non-adults, we find that we have not fitted about 62 million persons who are under age 18 years; we might even say we have as of this date largely given up on properly fitting (or safety restraining) our children.

Of course, NHTSA doesn't say anything like that, but they effectively do just that for child restraints by requiring only that the lap belt portion of a restraint fit a (six year-old) child, and they never do say what constitutes a "fit." Oh, what a "Federal Motor Vehicle Safety Standard" that is. See 49 CFR 571.208 S7 and 571.209 S4.1(g).

And this is more than a quarter of a century since this federal oversight organization, this protector of the automobile occupant, first went into business.

SUMMARY: THE VICTIM

We have now in rather general terms considered the victim, from the viewpoints of age, sex and habitus. We have found that there are profound changes of injury incidence and death rates as a function of age and sex, and that this is in part reflected in the breaking strengths of tissues.

We have also briefly touched on how size may effect the effectiveness of restraints by effecting fit of the restraints and, inferentially, by recalling some of the aspects of limited flail space discussed in the section on vehicles, how large people with maximal seated heights should have more, need more, flail volume. And inferentially,

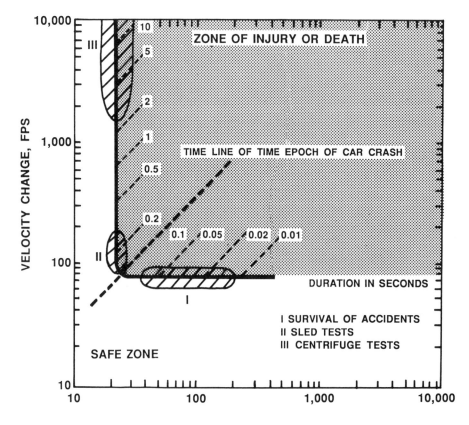

Figure 10
AN IMPACT SENSITIVITY CURVE FOR HUMAN BEINGS

This remarkable graphic representation of human tolerance to a wide range of acceleration stresses shows very many things, but it especially shows the uniqueness of the motor vehicle crash time epoch, occurring at the time-line labelled 0.1 seconds. Note that this time interval which characterizes motor vehicle crash occurs precisely at the break between the vertical line of tolerance for acceleration (here at about 20 G units) and the horizontal line of delta v (here at about 80 feet per second).

It says that, perhaps because we are just a bundle of tissues of differing viscoelasticities, we respond to *short duration impacts* (less than 0.1 second) only in terms of velocity changes (i.e., in terms of *delta v*) and to *long duration impacts* (greater than 0.1 second) primarily in terms of acceleration changes, (i.e., in terms of *G units*, or multiples of earth's gravitational pull).

It provides some feel for our biologic variation by the thickness of the scatter which forms each of the groups of tests. It also makes clear that even the apparently great biologic variation in acceleration tolerance is relatively small when compared to the overall time realm we are dealing with, that is, of durations from 0.01 seconds to 10 seconds, a range of a thousand-fold.

small drivers, in their need to reach the accelerator and brake pedals, may end up with their faces and chests quite close, too close, to the steering assembly.

All of which hopefully makes clear to the reader, even this early in the book, how variations in vehicle size and vehicle flail volumes may favorably or adversely interact with victim size, thereby either preventing or producing injury.

We will now end this long but hopefully not too arduous chapter with the last of the major crash factors.

THE VELOCITY

We have a rule here: for the average time epoch of a simple car crash, **the instantaneous change in velocity (delta v) is the best predictor of injury severity or death**[23][26][27][28].

However, the relationship between instantaneous change of velocity and injury severity (from the point of view of threat-to-life) is neither linear nor necessarily applicable to any one individual in any one crash. It is the *probability* of car occupant injury or death that increases with increasing delta v of the vehicle.

To a large degree, that is all that you need to know about velocity and injury or death.

Of course, "velocity" includes both speed and direction, and here we are discussing only the change in velocity in a scalar sense. We will deal with direction of impact and the principal direction of force in later portions of this book concerned with patterns of injury associated with various directions of impact: frontal, side, rear, etc.

For those readers who wish to know a bit more about velocity change and resultant injury of death, read on. For those readers without such interest, move on to chapter three, a crash course on how we break and tear what we are made of.

There appears to be a natural law in science that runs **many important papers first appear in obscure publications, but most papers in obscure publications are not important**. Many of the following references surely are obscure, but they are important.

The relationship between the change in velocity and the accelerative force exerted on a person is, to me at least, best described and understood by a curious derivative of a method originally developed by Kornhauser[29] at the Naval Ordinance Laboratory in White Oak, Maryland, in the mid-1940s, to describe the performance of ballistic devices such as impact switches. Twenty years later Kornhauser applied this same "impact sensitivity method" to animate beings, providing the basis for figure 10[30].

This figure plots the logarithm of delta v — as feet per second — against the logarithm of acceleration — as average G (average acceleration in multiples of earth's gravity. I know this all may appear to be opaque, but try to stay with me for just a moment more). The two thick lines at right angles to each other define rather clearly and simply that 20 average G and 80 feet per second velocity change must be exceeded for injury to occur to well restrained humans subject to accelerations transverse to their long axis.

Thus for an impact occurring in the time realm of about 100 milliseconds (i.e., 0.1 seconds), which is the time for a usual automotive crash and occurs in figure 10 at the lower left corner of the "Zone of Injury or Death," velocity changes less than about 80 feet per second and peak accelerations of 20 G or less (occurring for 100 milliseconds) are probably "safe," which is to say, survivable. Similarly, a 20 millisecond impact with a delta v below 80 feet per second is probably survivable even at 200 G. Or a 20 G accelerative load for 10 seconds is survivable even at velocity changes as great at 10,000 feet per second.

Although approximate, this is one of the most useful human tolerance graphs that I have encountered.

Don't stare at human tolerance tables too long, because they are not terribly useful unless they also represent the statistical variability that characterizes biology. Hard-line tolerance tables and curves in texts (generally without the points of data from which they were derived) do not always represent the biological variability that is in them, and therefore are not always quite as useful as they appear because they are not always sufficient. It's just that they are all that we have.

Remember that with regard to predicting injury or death, we generally can only measure the vehicle's velocity and the vehicle's change in velocity (delta v) during the crash; we rarely can obtain the occupant's delta v from the occupant's impact with the car's interior. With regard to vehicle delta v's, Danner's study of some 200 three-point seat belted drivers[26] showed that deaths did not occur until vehicle velocity changes of 65 kilometers per hour (about 40 miles per hour or nearly 60 feet per second), although serious to severe injuries (AIS 3,4) occurred at 50 to 70 kilometers per hour delta v (31 to 44 miles per hour). That was for the cars' velocity changes; we would expect the occupant contacts within the car that caused the fatal injuries to have velocity changes that may have been considerably higher.

Thus studies such as Danner's do not tell us that a vehicle delta v of 40 miles per hour in, say, a frontal collision will cause any one particular restrained occupant's death, only that we can expect *some* occupants to die at such a delta v, and that we can expect *more* deaths as the delta v increases.

BIBLIOGRAPHY

1. Occupant Death Rates, 1984-1988 Model Cars. *Status Report* Insurance Institute for Highway Safety, *26*:4, 1991.
2. Bazelon, D.T.: *The Paper Economy.* Vintage Books, New York, p. 198, 1965.
3. Fatal Accident Reporting System 1989, *NHTSA, DOT HS 807 693*, table 6-10, 1991.
4. Jones, I.S. and R.A. Whitfield: The effects of restraint use and mass in "downsized" cars. *SAE* paper 840199, 1984.
5. Partyka, S.: Car size trends in eleven years of fatal accidents. Math Analysis Div, Nat'l Ctr for Statistics and Analysis, *NHTSA, DOT,* April 1987.
6. Evans, L.: Car mass and likelihood of occupant fatality. *SAE* paper 820807, 1982.
7. Partyka, S., Sikora, J., Surti, J. and J. Van Dyke: Relative risk to car and light truck occupants. *SAE* paper 871093, 1987.
8. Partyka, S. and W.A. Boehly: Papers on car size: safety and trends. *NHTSA DOT HS* 807 444, June 1989.
9. Swearingen, J.J.: General aviation structures directly responsible for trauma in crash decelerations. *Dept. of Transportation, Office of Aviation Medicine,* Washington, D.C., 1971.
10. C.T. Morgan, A. Chapanis, J.S. Cook and M.W. Lund. (Eds.) *Human Engineering Guide to Equipment Design.* Table 11-13. McGraw-Hill Book Co., Inc., 1963.
11. Williams, A.F., Wong, J. and B.O'Neill: Occupant protection in interior impacts: an analysis of federal motor vehicle safety standard no. 201. *Proc 23rd Conf AAAM,* pp. 361-381, 1979.
12. Philippart, N.L., Kuechenmeister, T.J., Ferrara, R.A. and A.J. Arnold, Jr.: The effects of the steering wheel to pedal relationship on driver-selected seat position. *SAE* paper 850311, 1985.
13. Hackney, J.R., Hollowell, W.T. and D.S. Cohen: Analysis of frontal crash safety performance of passenger cars, light trucks and vans and an outline of future research requirements. *Proc 12th Int'l Tech Conf on Exptl Safety Vehicles,* table 5 p. 238, 1989. See also interior dimensions of vehicles in first 300 NCAP crash tests, 1989.

14. Dejeammes, M., Biard, R. and Y. Derrien: The three-point belt restraint: investigation of comfort needs, evaluation of efficacy improvements. *SAE* paper 840333, 1984.

15. Mitzkus, J.E. and H. Eyrainer: Three-point improvements for increased occupant protection. *SAE* paper 840395, 1984.

16. Armstrong, R.W. and H.P. Waters: Testing programs and research on restraint systems. *SAE* paper 690247, 1969.

17. Robertson, L.S.: *Injuries: causes, control strategies and public policy.* Lexington Books, Lexington p. 9, 1983.

18. Baker, S.P., O'Neill, B. and R.S. Karpf: *The injury fact book.* Lexington Books, Lexington p. 195, 1984.

19. Fife, D., Barancik, J.I. and B.F. Chatterjee: Northeastern Ohio trauma study II: injury rates by age, sex and cause. *Am J Public Health 74*:5, p. 473-478, May 1984.

20. Partyka, S.C., Letter, June 16, 1989.

21. van Kampen, L.T.B.: Traffic accidents of elderly people in the Netherlands; they really are more vulnerable than other road users. *Proc 12th Int'l Tech Conf on Exptl Safety Vehicles*, pp. 85-91, 1989.

22. Evans, L.: Risk of fatality from physical trauma versus sex and age. *J Trauma 28*:3, pp. 368-378, 1988.

23. Malliaris, A.C., Hitchcock, R. and M. Hansen: Harm causation and ranking in car crashes. *SAE* paper 850090, 1985.

24. Nachemson, A.L., Schultz, A.B. and M.H. Berkson: Mechanical properties of human lumbar spine segments: influences of age, sex, disc level and degeneration. *Spine 4*:1 pp. 1-8, 1979.

25. Yamada, H.: *Strength of biological materials.* (Ed. by F.G. Evans) Williams and Wilkins, Baltimore p. 75-80, 1970.

26. Danner, M., Langwieder, D. and T. Hummel: The effect of restraint systems and possibilities of future improvements derived from real-life accidents. *SAE* paper 840394, 1984.

27. Langwieder, K., Danner, M., Schmelzing, W., Appel, H., Kramer, F. and J. Hoffman: Comparison of passenger injuries in frontal car collisions with dummy loadings in equivalent simulations. *SAE* paper 791009, 1979.

28. Foust, D.R., Bowan, B.M. and R.G. Snyder: Study of human impact tolerance using investigations and simulations of free falls. *SAE* paper 770915, 1977.

29. Kornhauser, M.: Prediction and evaluation of sensitivity to transient accelerations. *J Appl Mech 21*:371, 1954.
30. Kornhauser, M. and A. Gold: Application of the impact sensitivity method to animate structures. *Nat Acad Sc/Nat Res Council* publication 977 p. 333-344, 1962.

CHAPTER 3

HOW WE BREAK AND TEAR THE STUFF WE ARE MADE OF

(i.e., Biomechanics Revisited)

GENERAL

According to Keith L. Moore[1], "Anatomy students learn a new language consisting of at least 4500 words." This is not too surprising; the classical text *Gray's Anatomy* opens with: "The entire skeleton in the adult consists of 200 distinct bones." And that's just bones. The bones connect to another 220 or so muscles. We are not even going to mention the arteries, veins, nerves, organs and the tissues that compose organs.

And we also add lots more names when we break bones. According to *The Fracture Classification Manual*[2], there are 20 different fractures classified just for collar bone (clavicle) fractures, even without such sub-classes as open or closed, or displaced or undisplaced. And for the thigh bone (femur) the Manual names 42 fractures without delving into the fracture-dislocations that would add at least another 20 named femoral fractures.

There was a saying in medical school that "Every department wants to teach their course last." That is, it is much easier to teach medical concepts when the student is both versed and at least somewhat experienced in anatomy, physiology, biochemistry, pathology, etc. What I'm getting at is: there is no way that I can give you in brief the detail that it would be nice for you to know. Having now provided you with two anatomy references and a fracture manual, I can here only give you an overview, and a much simplified one at that, of what we are made of, from the lowly placed viewpoint of one cell talking about another.

WHAT ARE WE MADE OF?

In our teens, about 60 percent water, by weight. By age sixty or so we fatten up enough to be about 50 percent water. (Fat cells have almost no water in them, so as our fat content goes up, our percentage water content goes down.)

Some 5 percent of our body weight is the water in blood plasma; about 15 percent is in the fluid outside of our cells and outside of our blood vessels, the fluid that bathes our cells that we call "interstitial" fluid. The remaining 40 percent of our body weight that is water is found inside of the aggregate of cells we call "us" and which we term "intracellular fluid."

So we are made of cells, and the cells of which we are made are largely water and are themselves bathed by a watery fluid outside of the cells and outside of the blood vessels.

How many cells are we made of?

Well, estimates vary, but about a hundred million body cells or so, with an average size of a hundredth of a millimeter in diameter, at least according to one anatomy atlas[3]. But that must not count the central nervous system, which would add another trillion or so neurons (functional cells of the nervous system) and 10 to 50 trillion glial cells[4] (i.e., neuroglial cells, of which there are four distinct cell types serving as the connective tissue of the nervous system). And that clearly does not count circulating red blood cells, of which there are about 3 times 10 to the thirteenth power, or some thirty thousand trillion cells circulating[4].

All of our cells vary enormously in shape, size and what they do for a living. Nerve cells (neurons), for example, concentrate on the transmission of electrical signals. Muscle cells are specially made to lengthen and shorten on signal, thus creating motion. And there are hundreds of other cell types, each specialized for one or more functions.

So it appears that we are made of millions and millions of cells which themselves appear to be largely made up of water, rather like small bags of non-homogeneous gelatin, or very, very small jelly fish. The question is, why don't these millions of tiny bags of gelatin simply fall apart from each other and roll across the floor?

I guess we would do just that if the cells weren't somehow held together.

In order then to understand how we break and tear we must first have *some* idea how cells attach to each other and what holds cells together in the cell-aggregates we call "tissues," and in the tissue-aggregates we call "organs."

HOW WE KEEP FROM COMING APART

There are two quite different junctions between cells, types that actually fasten cells to each other and to surrounding tissues ("tight junctions") and types that allow for molecules and ions to exchange between cells (the so-called "gap junctions").

Cells are fastened to each other by some four different kinds of fastenings, but I doubt much clarity will come to us by seeing their names, to wit: zonula occludens, zonula adherens, desmosomes and hemidesmosomes.

The zonula occludens (no, you don't have to learn these names; I'm just trying to give you a feel for the subject) is a "tight junction," a broad band of ridges of contact between cells; the zonula adherens and hemidesmosomes seem to be smaller, patchy areas of junction, and desmosomes appear as simple small points of attachment.

There also are certain adhesive proteins that literally glue certain tissue cells together. Finally, there are materials produced by specialized cells that remain outside of cells, providing a matrix to support and bind cells together within the matrix. This extracellular matrix also provides strength and elasticity to the cell-aggregate, the tissue.

Examples of matrix material would include such viscous and jelly-like substances as hyaluronic acid and chondroitin. But the matrix substances that are most ubiquitous are fibrous and elastic support fibers, the former made primarily of a unique protein called "collagen," and the latter made of a protein called "elastin," which, unsurprisingly, is quite elastic.

By virtue of its great tensile strength (i.e., resistance to being pulled apart), collagen is of itself largely responsible for the mechanical strength of soft connective tissue. Weight for weight, when put into tension, collagen fibers are about as strong as steel[5]. These fibers of collagen are most often imbedded in other matrices outside of cells, and are in a sense similar to the fiberglass fibers set in a polyester medium in the material from which we manufacture such items as modern boats, termed "fiberglass reinforced plastic."

It is the collagen fibers, the elastic fibers and the reticular fibers, all different, thread-like fibers imbedded in mineral, gelatinous, and adhesive matrices that form our bones, cartilage, tendons, ligaments, as well as the reticulum and elastic fibers that support our blood vessels, nerves, muscle fibers and the like. These are our connective tissues, and collagen is their mainstay, constituting approximately one-third of all of the protein in our entire bodies[6].

There are ten quite different connective tissues, but I'll not list them all here. It should be sufficient that by now you have some sort of picture of our intercellular

INJURY MECHANISMS

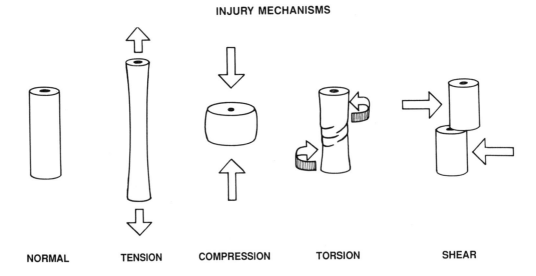

NORMAL   TENSION   COMPRESSION   TORSION   SHEAR

(DISPLACEMENTS SHOWN ARE SCHEMATIC AND EXAGGERATED)

Figure 11
DIRECTIONS OF THE FORCES THAT TEAR US APART

This illustration shows a viscoelastic thick-walled cylinder subjected to *all* of the possible directions by which force may be applied to it. The forces being exerted here are called *stresses*.

The responses of the cylinder here are both exaggerated and schematic, in the name of clarity. The response to the forces/stresses are displacements, and we call them *strains*.

I hope that these simple stresses and the resultant strains are *very clear* to you, because they are, in large part, the basis of understanding how and why we break and tear the way we do.

TENSION = to pull apart
COMPRESSION = to push together
TORSION = to twist (or wring)
SHEAR = to slide apart (in opposite but parallel directions)

Strain is the displacement that is caused by a stress.

**BENDING FORCE APPLIED
TO THICK WALLED CYLINDER (SEE TEXT)**

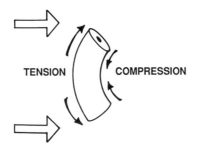

TENSION   COMPRESSION

Figure 12
BENDING FORCES

Long bones, such as our thigh bones, will not infrequently be fractured by bending forces.

This illustration is intended to show that bending, as applied to a thick walled cylinder (or a long bone), is made up of tension on one side of the cylinder and of compression on the other side of the cylinder.

**COMBINED TORSION AND COMPRESSION
APPLIED TO THICK WALLED CYLINDER**

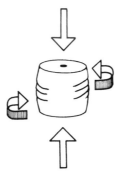

Figure 13
COMPRESSION AND TORSION COMBINED . . .

. . . and applied to a thick walled cylinder.

This illustrates that any number of forces (stresses) may be applied together to cause a combination of displacements (strains) that would not ordinarily occur *unless* they were caused by combined stresses.

The lesson to be learned here is that unusual and extraordinary fractures and tears of softer tissues should cause us to seek unusual and extraordinary combinations of forces that could have caused them.

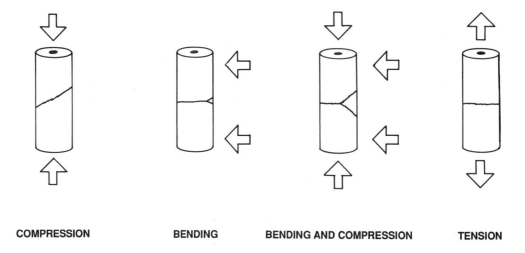

| COMPRESSION | BENDING | BENDING AND COMPRESSION | TENSION |

Figure 14
TYPICAL FRACTURE PATTERNS IN THE MIDPORTION OF A LONG BONE

By subjecting a long bone (femur, humerus, tibia, etc.) to some of the stresses typical of crashes we may see characteristic fracture patterns in the long bone.

Note the *oblique* fracture shown above due to compression, the *transverse* fracture with what is termed a *butterfly fragment* at the convex side that results from bending (and a typically much larger version of the butterfly fragment that results from combined bending and compression). Simple tension causes a purely *transverse* fracture, seen in the right side of this rather idealized representation of long bone fractures.

Fracture patterns generally are so characteristic of the forces (stresses) that caused them that they usually permit us to define the directions of the force(s) that caused them.

You may also want to consider that a fracture is simply a strain (displacement) caused by a stress (force) that exceeded the *elasticity* of the material of which the long bone is composed. In a sense, this is not unlike subjecting a rubber band (a very elastic material) to progressive tension (i.e., stretching the rubber band) until the rubber band's elastic limit was exceeded, which is to say that the rubber band was stretched until it broke.

fastening systems and of their surprising complexity, of how we are held together and why our cells don't fall apart and skitter across the floor like millions of microscopic beads.

You should visualize that we are held together by: multiple mechanical fastenings between adjacent cells; additional extra-cellular glues (adhesives) imbedding cell groups; fibrous surrounds of elastic and other fibers; and extra-cellular mineral deposits entirely encapsulating cells, as in bone.

For most tissues we find that we are held together so well that a considerable force is needed to tear us apart.

FORCES THAT TRY TO TEAR US APART

We need to know three things about the forces that would tear us to pieces: 1) we need know the directions they take, and 2) we need know how such forces are measured and the units by which they are measured and reported to us in journals and handbooks. In order to understand why a given force will sometimes tear us asunder and at other times the same magnitude of force will not do so, we also need to know of a third thing, 3) the tissue property called "visco-elasticity," why some mechanical properties of connective tissues change with different rates of applying loads (force), why these properties are "time dependent."

To illustrate what directions of forces would pull us apart, we will take a hollow section of a thick walled, relatively plastic cylinder and subject it to forces in different directions, showing in an exaggerated fashion the deformations caused by the forces; see figure 11.

The forces exerted upon the bone segments are termed stresses.

The deformations caused by stresses are termed strains.

The stress-strain relationship — how much stress causes how much strain — (or how much force causes how much deformation) — is a key relationship graphically describing any given material, including complex materials such as bone or ligament.

Looking at figure 11 we see that there are only four modes of loading, four directions of force: tension, compression, torsion and shear. Figure 12 shows that bending is really not another, separate mode; rather, it may be considered that the tubular section is subject to tension on one side (convex) and to compression on the other (concave) side.

In the real world of trauma it is rare that a pure load is applied; instead, a limb (here a deformable cylinder) may be concurrently subjected to compression with torsion (figure 13), or other combinations of loads, as in figure 14, which shows how compression plus bending when carried to structural failure will cause quite typical patterns of fracture. Let me emphasize that the fracture patterns that result from such forces are generally so characteristic of the forces that caused them that we often can and do rely on such patterns to reconstruct what must have happened to a given occupant in a given accident.

The measure of forces shown in figures 11 to 14 is generally given in units of force, termed "Newtons" (N). To anyone who has not taken Physics 102-a in college ("Good heavens, my degree was in International Affairs! Why would I take Physics?"), to such an individual these units of force could be Martian. But go along with me for just a little while; it will cause neither pain nor permanent disability.

Sir Isaac Newton's second law of motion states that when a particle free to move is subject to a force, the particle (or body) will accelerate in a fashion proportional to the force and inversely proportional to its own mass. Or,

$$force = mass \times acceleration$$

Force has dimensions of mass (say, kilograms, or kg) multiplied by the dimensions of acceleration (say, meters per second per second, or m/s/s). Or,

$$1 \text{ Newton (a unit of force)} = 1 \text{ kg} \times 1 \text{ m/s/s}$$

Similarly, the unit of pressure (and stress) is termed a Pascal (Pa), and is given as

$$1 \text{ Pa} = 1 \text{ Newton per 1 square meter.}$$

All of this simple but mathematical-looking stuff really is necessary in order to discuss things such as stress, (which we now know may be measured in units called "Pascals," or Pa, and is simply a measure of force-per-unit-area, which, in the metric system, could be reported as Newtons per square meter). Later in this chapter, when we actually use this sort of information, I will convert the "Newtons per square meter" to "pounds per square inch," since we all should have some idea of what a pound feels like and what a square inch looks like.

Finally, before putting all of this together to make some sort of grand picture, we need to understand that what we are mostly made of may be termed as "visco-elastic" material by people who would use such terminology, such as an engineer, or even a biophysicist.

THROW SILLY PUTTY AND IT BOUNCES

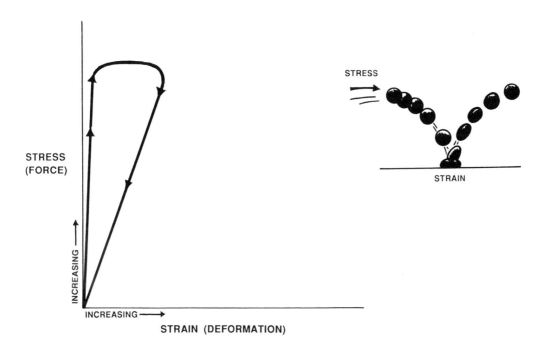

Figure 15
VISCOELASTICITY

Here, using Silly Putty, a silicone plastic that is the most viscoelastic material that I know of, we illustrate its elasticity by a stress/strain graph (to the left), and by a cartoon (to the right side).

We see that a rapidly applied stress will cause the material to quickly deform and then quickly return to about its original shape.

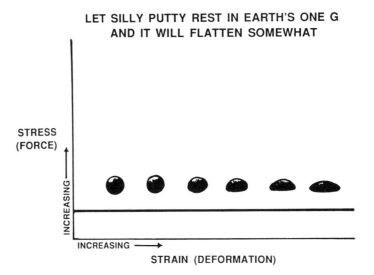

Figure 16
VISCOELASTICITY

Here's another graph with a cartoon. This one shows an exaggerated response, the viscous or "slow flow" of the Silly Putty subject to a constant stress (the force of gravity).

To describe it properly, we see deformation (strain) resulting from a constant stress (gravity).

The proper term for a change in deformation which results from a constant stress is "*creep*", but we will not deal with either creep or the change in stress that results from constant deformation — which is properly termed *stress relaxation* — because I believe such terms have caused acute bladder spasm in some who prefer arts to the sciences.

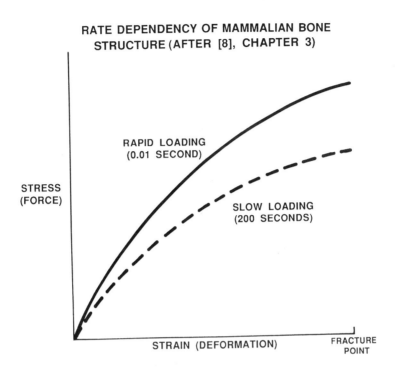

RATE DEPENDENCY OF MAMMALIAN BONE
STRUCTURE (AFTER [8], CHAPTER 3)

STRESS
(FORCE)

RAPID LOADING
(0.01 SECOND)

SLOW LOADING
(200 SECONDS)

STRAIN (DEFORMATION)   FRACTURE
                          POINT

Figure 17
THE RATE DEPENDENCY OF MAMMALIAN BONE

This graph is presented for those who prefer graphs to words. It shows that bones may sustain without breaking a higher force rapidly applied and withdrawn than they may sustain when even a lower force is more slowly applied.

A simple example would be if you jumped off a table and landed in a rather flat-footed fashion. It would be a jolt, but I doubt that anything within you would break, because it all happened and was over so fast that there was not much time for tissues to be displaced.

What happened? Why, the jolt was about 30 G. Everything within you was *very briefly* subject to a force about 30 times that of Earth's gravity, but it was all over in *thousandths* of a second.

However, if the 30 G force was sustained for a while, say a few seconds, chances are that something within you would break. Why would it break? Well, if you weigh 150 pounds, then at 30 G you would have the virtual weight of 2.25 *tons*, and, as I said, chances are something within you would break under that load when prolonged. For example, static axial compression of the femur will fracture the shaft of that bone at under 1,800 pounds of load (O. Messerer in 1880, and W.R. Powell et al in 1975, reported in ref. 13, chapter 3).

> *viscoelasticity* = a property of a material whereby a change of stress occurs under constant deformation (termed "stress relaxation"), or, a change in deformation occurs under constant load (termed "creep").

Fortunately, this esoteric definition, derived from an excellent basic biomechanics text[7], is best clarified with that most marvelous material, Silly Putty, which is about as viscoelastic as anything can get.

If I throw a ball of Silly Putty against the floor it will bounce right back up to me and I'll not even find a flat spot on it where it contacted the floor. (I know this is so because I just got up from my word processor, found my trusty ball of Silly Putty in my desk drawer, rolled it into a round ball and threw it against my ceramic tile floor.) It is as elastic as a rubber ball. But if I slowly squeeze the stuff between thumb and forefinger, (and I'm doing just that right now!), it flattens and assumes a biconcave configuration and stays that way. Similarly, if I *slowly* draw the Silly Putty apart, I can form a string two or three feet long; if I try to do so rapidly, the Silly Putty abruptly breaks into two pieces.

These exaggerated viscoelastic properties of Silly Putty are represented in figures 15, 16 and 17, although figure 17 uses bone rather than Silly Putty to make the point.

Playing with this putty is not as silly as it seems; the viscoelastic properties of our connective tissues may well determine whether we live or die in a given impact, whether an aorta, for example, simply stretches or whether it tears; whether a chest sustains fatal or less-than-fatal injury on impact. In short, whether a tissue breaks apart when suddenly pulled (as did the Silly Putty) or whether it stretches viscously or whether we elastically deform and spring back to shape (as also did the Silly Putty) may well *depend on the rate at which the force is exerted upon the tissue*, will depend upon the time-epoch, (as it did with the Silly Putty).

Viscoelasticity is a property of all tissues. Even hard tissues such as bone will break under different loads in a time-dependent, rate-of-application-of-force-dependent, fashion[8], see also figure 17.

Now if you return to the definition of viscoelasticity given above, it may well have become more intelligible, because playing with Silly Putty can make it so.

SOME TISSUES AND THEIR MECHANICAL TOLERANCES

In order to get some sort of feeling for what does or does not exist in the hand-books of impact tolerance and in biomechanics review articles and, more importantly, how useful and practical such information may be, we will give Donald Driver, a 65 year old male driver of a small car, a diagonal 2 inch by one-half inch deep laceration of his right temple and forehead. That's where Donald Driver struck the steering wheel rim with his forehead. He also fractured his right cheek bone (zygoma) when he struck his right forearm with the right side of his face, without breaking either the skin of the cheek, the skin of the forearm or the bones of the forearm. The zygomatic fracture is a simple fracture (e.g., broken into two pieces) and it is a closed fracture (i.e., does not communicate to the outer surface of the skin). These are unremarkable crash injuries.

What reference books and tables contain information about how much force it takes to tear the skin of the forehead and how much force should it take to break the cheekbone (zygoma)? The skin and zygoma of a sixty-five year old male, that is.

Since the Society of Automotive Engineers provides handbooks of such information that should be the basis for motor vehicle design, as well as what the SAE also terms "SAE Ground Vehicle Standards," we will turn to the SAE handbooks, the publications **SAE J885 JUL86[9] and SAE J202[10]**, the latter being an "SAE Information Report" referenced in the former publication as "the state-of-the-art in assessing skin injuries."

I guess that I felt compelled to put these references in bold type and underline them because they appear to be the source material for automotive design from the viewpoint of human tolerance to crash forces; witness that these publications were developed by the SAE "HUMAN INJURY CRITERIA TASK FORCE" composed of one member from Chrysler, one from NHTSA, one from Wayne State University, two from General Motors and two from Ford Motor Company.

So in SAE J885 we find, in section 3.4 ("Biomechanical Materials"), sub-section 3.4.2 ("soft tissues"), under 3.4.2.1, "Skin," that "Skin has been studied more than any other soft tissue insofar as automotive collision trauma is concerned." We are then referred to "the state-of-the-art in assessing skin injuries" summarized in SAE Information Report J202.

Report J202 is about 2/3rds of a page. It has no data at all about what forces are necessary to lacerate skin. It offers "materials that are currently employed in automotive testing laboratories to simulate human skin," to wit: 1) Chamois, 2) PPG formulation (a sponge rubber base covered with an RTV silicone rubber and impregnated with human hair) and 3) Inland skin and flesh, a composite headform covering developed for automotive hardware testing (see SAE 690746, May 1969).

Well, it is clear that the SAE will not help us to find the force necessary to cause a 2' x 1/2" laceration on the scalp of a 65 year old man, our good friend Donald

Driver, so we will look elsewhere, to the Japanese Automobile Research Institute "Handbook of Human Tolerance," which was written by three Americans[11]. This fine text provides us with graphic data (figure 2-58) for skin in front of and behind the ear (not quite forehead, but close) which ranges from 1,000 to 2,000 lbs per square inch. We also see that the tensile breaking strength of skin at age 60-69 is .7 that of age 30-49 (table 2-34), so we can estimate the tensile strength at .7 x 1,000-2,000 lbs/square inch, or 700 to 1,400 lbs/square inch. Correcting for the size of the laceration and making certain assumptions — such as the tensile strength being close to the shear and compressive strength of skin (which it may or may not be), we can come up with at least some sort of an estimate.

And what does it take to simply break a zygoma?

Here SAE J885 provides us with some help, under 4.3 "Strength of Facial Bones." Subsection 4.3.1 is "Zygoma," and it references four available studies, each of which used padded impactors from about 1 and 1/8th inches to about 2 and 1/2 inches in diameter. Fortunately, they all gave *about* the same tolerance, from about 250 to 525 lbs.

With an average male head weighing in at about 9.1 pounds, (we'll call it 10 lbs because it's easier to work with and this whole exercise appears to be a rough calculation at best), we can estimate that Donald Driver's head struck the combined surfaces of his right forearm and the right upper steering wheel rim with about 700 to 1,000 lbs of force, which could then both break his cheekbone and cause a 2 inch or so laceration of his forehead. His head (which we estimated at about 10 lbs) had to have a virtual weight then of 1/4 to 1/2 ton, which is to say his head struck the steering assembly and forearm at about 70 to 100 G. This is not unreasonable; it is in fact typical for the dummy driver's head to strike the steering assembly with about 275 G's in the NHTSA New Car Assessment Program, a 35 mile per hour frontal barrier crash test (!).

So Donald Driver's injuries could have been incurred in a 20 to 30 mile per hour "barrier equivalent speed" accident — about a 20 to 30 mph delta v — while fully restrained by a three point restraint system.

Anyone for air bags?

HUMAN TOLERANCE TO INJURY: (OR, THE GREAT BIOMECHANICS ILLUSION)

What is a science?

In its youth, a science is largely classificatory; the measurements taken within the area of study permitting grouping of diverse phenomena.

As the science matures, measurable properties can be mathematically related and systematic theories can be constructed. When the science has fully matured, the theoretic principles permit prediction of what will happen under specific conditions, and predictions can then be made and their accuracy validated by tests.

The truth is, I can think of no truly unifying theory within the entire field that we call "biomechanics." There isn't even a generally accepted unitary or even unifying theory of human tolerance to accelerative force, and here I mean to all six degrees of freedom of motion.

Perhaps the best attempt at unifying multi-directional human impact tolerance theory known to me is that of Payne's[12]. His work, more of a combined overview and grouping of unifying theories, is still the closest thing to a series of unifying theories that we have. It was done under contract to the U.S. Air Force in 1984, was never either published by the USAF or released for independent publication, for reasons still unclear to me.

The last (1986) edition of the Society of Automotive Engineer's "Human Tolerance to Impact Conditions as Related to Motor Vehicle Design" (SAE J885)[9], is, in and of itself, an indication of our presently inadequate biomechanical basis for automotive safety design. It is about 70 pages long, has 3 figures and 14 tables. Most of what is listed on the tables requires text for explanation, partly because the tests of any two investigators generally are not directly comparable, one using an impactor of one dimension, another using an impactor of another dimension, and so forth. In short, little has been standardized in the way of either tests or methods of reporting test results by the appropriate learned societies. A more complete and more useful as well as more recent review of human response to impact stress (of research published through 1984) is that of Melvin and Weber[13], while the most complete Handbook of Human Tolerance was published by the Japan Automobile Research Institute (!), written by three Americans (!!!)[11] some sixteen years ago, and required 631 pages, even then, in 1976. (The inference, that no U.S. institution — federal, corporate or societal — chose to sponsor this publication at that time, is appalling if true.)

In the preface to the Japanese publication, one of the authors, J.H. McElhaney, aptly noted that the field of biomechanics of trauma is like the field of celestial mechanics before the time of Keppler, which is to say that present biomechanics of trauma has "a multitude of measurements and experimental data, but no unifying theories that allow extrapolation to new situations[11]."

This was still true eleven years later, in 1987, when SAE J885 was published, and remains true today.

In 1987, what was termed a "Government/Industry Meeting and Exposition" was held in Washington, D.C. The biomechanics of injury was presented as it was being studied in some 32 laboratories throughout the western world[14]. The disparate efforts were both emphasized and contrasted by Dr. David Viano (of GM Research Laboratories) who urged that the attendees, should "establish a science of biomechanics. Rather than answer specific questions, answer them in the broader framework; development of principles so that we can legitimize the field." He said also that "biomechanics deals with the application of scientific principles to the human; the human's reaction to force. And, although it is difficult for us to evaluate the human in severe exposures and we resort to doing dummy testing, animal modeling or cadaver work, *the whole purview of the field could be advanced if we legitimize it into a professional science.*" (The emphasis is mine).

What Dr. Viano, a practicing and productive biomechanicist was saying both more eloquently and more believably than most, is that for all practical purposes, at this time in history *there may not be a legitimate existing science that we can call "Biomechanics,"* that if we look to larger principles, to general theories of human impact tolerance, there are no such things extant. All we have is a morass of data, variously obtained and only occasionally or by chance alone comparable to other data.

We have attempted to develop and use mathematical and mechanical models in the looming absence of an adequate standard data base by which we could validate the models. We are still attempting to put theoretic model carts before valid data base horses.

It is nevertheless worth perusing what data we do have, looking for a reasonable fit to a particular situation, which is why I have written of the way such data is reported and where much of it is summarized and available. It is often worth perusing what data we do have, but it is also at least as often not worth the perusal, because we so often find that we cannot extrapolate from the data found.

At this point in time I believe that Biomechanics is more of a promise than a fact, the presence of Biomechanics Journals, Biomechanics Societies and university based Biomechanics Departments now granting doctoral degrees in Biomechanics — all of these trappings of a legitimate science not withstanding.

So much for the state of the art in Biomechanics in the early 1990s.

SUMMARY

We have attempted to gain insight into how our cells and tissues are held together and how they are torn apart. We have seen how the viscoelasticity of our tissues makes them, to some degree, time dependent in how they respond to a given force. That is, the same amount and direction of force may cause irrevocable damage if applied in one time period and may cause no significant harm if applied in another, say slower, fashion. And for some other tissues, the reverse may be true.

Using two specific and relatively trivial injuries — that of torn skin of the forehead and a broken cheek bone — we have looked up the sort of forces that are necessary to cause these injuries. We found biomechanics source handbooks to be both quite variable, and difficult to apply to any one singular, common, crash event.

We then looked to the young field of Biomechanics and found to our deep regret a very large amount of data, much of it not relatable to other data, and essentially devoid of the general theories and explanations that would permit generalization and extrapolation.

We found, in short, a science still largely without the general laws necessary to build upon.

We will hope that, as the field of study grows older, it will also grow appropriately mature, that it will ultimately fulfill its great promise and will actually provide, among other things, a sound basis for injury reduction by sound designs based on sound predictions of tissue damage thresholds.

BIBLIOGRAPHY

1. Moore, K.L.: *Clinically Oriented Anatomy*. 2nd Ed., Williams & Wilkins, Baltimore p.3, 1985.
2. Gustilo, R.B.: *The Fracture Classification Manual*. Mosby Year Book, St. Louis, 1991.
3. *Atlas of Anatomy*. Marshall Cavendish Books, Ltd., London p.18, 1990.
4. Ganong, W.F.: *Review of Medical Physiology*. 15th Ed., Appleton & Lange, Norwalk p.43, 1991.
5. *Ibid.*, p. 362.
6. White, A., Handler, P. and E.L. Smith: *Principles of Biochemistry*. McGraw-Hill, New York, 1964.
7. Nordin, M. and V.H. Frankel: *Basic Biomechanics of the Musculoskeletal System*. 2nd Ed., Lea & Febiger, Phila. p. 309, 1989.
8. Ibid., p. 17; Sammarco, J., Burstein, A., Davis, W. and V. Frankel: The biomechanics of torsional fractures: the effect of loading on ultimate properties. *J Biomech 4*:113, 1971.
9. *Human Tolerance to Impact Conditions As Related to Motor Vehicle Design*. SAE *J885*, July 1986.
10. *Synthetic Skins for Automotive Testing*. SAE *J202*, 1972.
11. McElhaney, J.H., Roberts, V.L. and J.F. Hilyard: *Handbook of Human Tolerance*. Japan Automobile Research Institute, Inc., Tokyo, 1976.
12. Payne, P.R.: Linear and angular short duration acceleration allowables for the human body. *KTR 357-84*, USAF Contract F33615-81-0500, 1984.
13. Melvin, J.W. and K. Weber (eds.): Review of biomechanical impact response and injury in the automotive environment. *DOT HS 807 042*; also SAE *B-523*, 1987.
14. *Injury Biomechanics*. SAE *SP-731*, 1987.

CHAPTER 4

WHEREIN WE DEFINE, DESCRIBE AND DAMAGE MUSCLES, BONES AND JOINTS

GENERAL

This chapter is concerned with characteristic musculoskeletal crash injuries. References[1] [2] [3] [4] are three recommended anatomy texts and an atlas, although most any anatomy text or atlas would probably suffice.

As we noted from Donald Driver's injuries in chapter 3, it is possible to break a bone without lacerating the overlying skin. We call such fractures **closed fractures**. Immediately after fracturing a bone, in fact, except for an occasional deformity such as swelling, the skin overlying most fractures gives little or no indication at all of the injury below!

Of course, when the fracture site communicates to the outside of the skin, it is known as an **open fracture**, and, from my experience, it usually is a sight at least as appalling as is the injury and its consequences.

The fracture of Donald Driver's cheekbone you will recall, took about 500 lbs (per square inch), but lacerating the nearby skin of his forehead took more than twice that force per square inch, meaning that the **force necessary to break some bones may be much less than that necessary to tear some skin**.

From the somewhat morbid viewpoint of injury causation analyses, broken bones and damaged joints are analytic conveniences, radiographically offering evidence of directions and approximate magnitudes of the forces that caused them; recall figure 14 in chapter 3, and also see table 3, in this chapter. Skeletal damage generally is of great use in reconstructing occupant motion or trajectories.

Skin bruises, abrasions and lacerations are important and useful too, but generally are less helpful then are the muscle, joint and skeletal injuries. For one thing, the tissue just beneath the overlying skin (the dermis and epidermis) but above the fascial cover of muscle, a loose and relatively weak, elastic layer containing variable amounts of fat cells, nerves and blood vessels — called "subcutaneous tissue" — is much more readily damaged than is the overlying skin. This is especially so for the

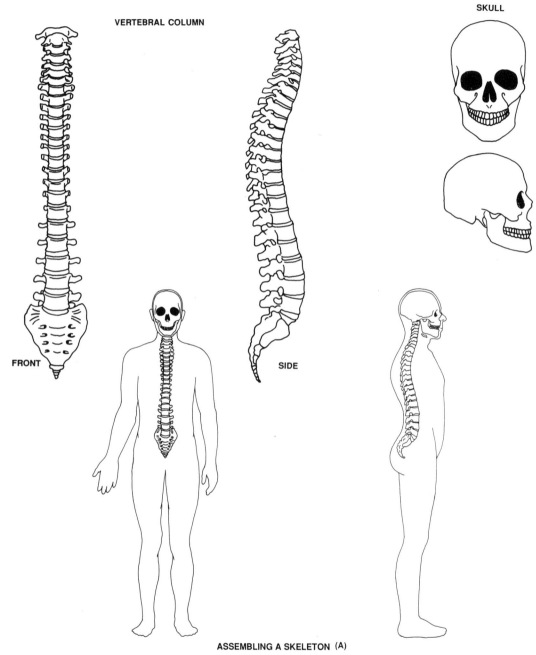

VERTEBRAL COLUMN

SKULL

FRONT

SIDE

ASSEMBLING A SKELETON (A)

Figure 18
THE AXIAL (LOAD-BEARING) SKELETON

Here we place a head on top of the spinal column (18A), engage the base of the bony spine into the pelvis (18B) and hook up the lower extremities into the pelvis by the ball-and-socket joint of the hip (18C), thereby creating the *weight-bearing skeleton.*

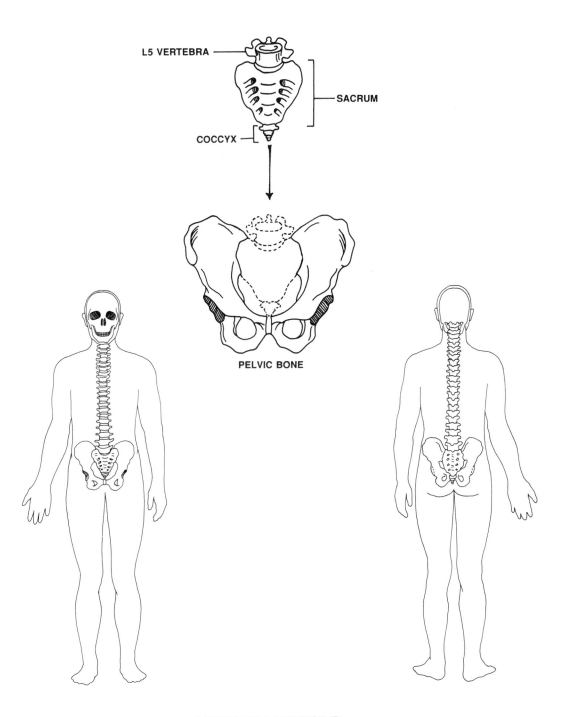

L5 VERTEBRA

SACRUM

COCCYX

PELVIC BONE

ASSEMBLING A SKELETON (B)

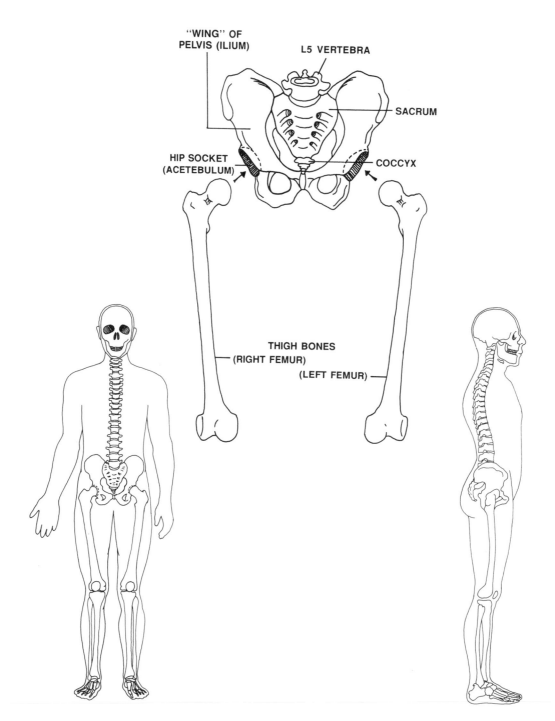

"WING" OF
PELVIS (ILIUM)

L5 VERTEBRA

SACRUM

HIP SOCKET
(ACETEBULUM)

COCCYX

THIGH BONES
(RIGHT FEMUR)
(LEFT FEMUR)

ASSEMBLING A SKELETON (C)

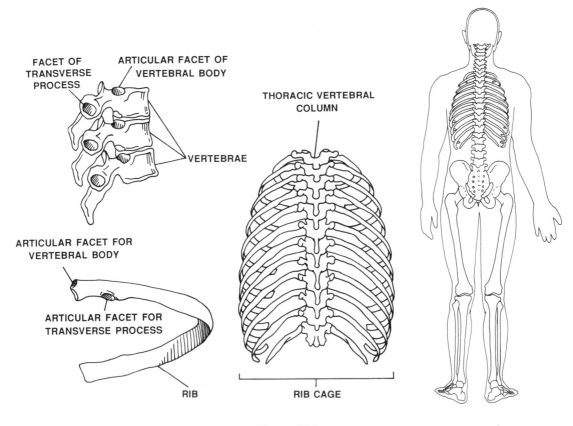

FACET OF TRANSVERSE PROCESS

ARTICULAR FACET OF VERTEBRAL BODY

VERTEBRAE

ARTICULAR FACET FOR VERTEBRAL BODY

ARTICULAR FACET FOR TRANSVERSE PROCESS

RIB

THORACIC VERTEBRAL COLUMN

RIB CAGE

Figure 19A

Figure 19 A, B, C
ASSEMBLY OF THE ENTIRE SKELETON, BOTH AXIAL AND NON-LOAD BEARING MEMBERS

In order to assemble the entire skeleton we have to add to the axial (i.e., weight-bearing) skeleton of figure 18 the additional bones of the: ribs and sternum (19A), the collar bones and shoulder blades (19B), and the upper extremities (19C).

Note that the upper extremities connect to the axial skeleton only at the collar bones (clavicles), where they attach to the breast bone (the sternum), while the remainder of the upper extremities attach only to muscles, not at all directly to other bones.

This distinction, between load bearing and non-load bearing skeletons and of how they attach to each other, is being made to so that we may better understand what groups of bones may be injured by *transmitted forces* and what bones may be damaged only by *direct forces* applied to them.

Figure 19B

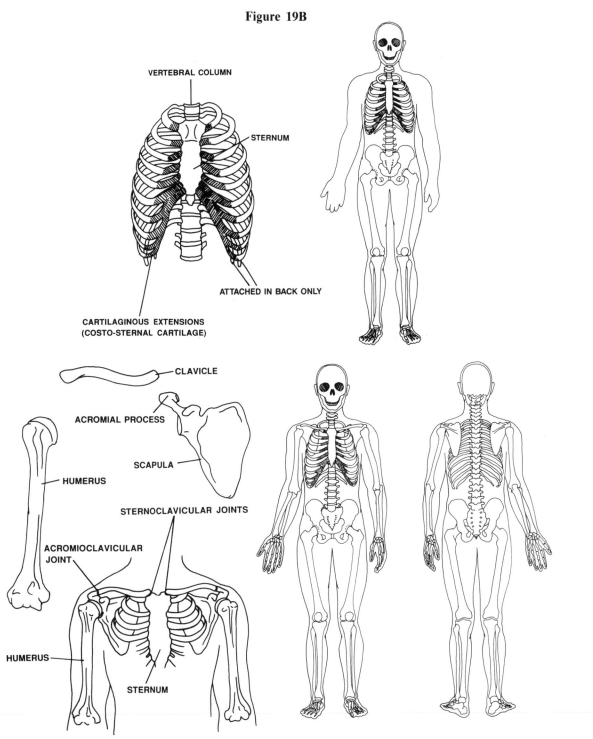

VERTEBRAL COLUMN

STERNUM

ATTACHED IN BACK ONLY

CARTILAGINOUS EXTENSIONS
(COSTO-STERNAL CARTILAGE)

CLAVICLE

ACROMIAL PROCESS

SCAPULA

HUMERUS

STERNOCLAVICULAR JOINTS

ACROMIOCLAVICULAR
JOINT

HUMERUS

STERNUM

Figure 19C

blood vessels contained in the subcutaneous tissue, and we therefore get a lot of bleeding into the subcutaneous layer.

Both clinically and in our individual experiences we have seen apparently undamaged skin with substantial bleeding below it. The subcutaneous bleeding first is manifest by swelling, then later is followed by discoloration of the overlying skin as the blood spilled into the subcutaneous tissue from torn blood vessels dissects outward, into the dermis, causing what we then recognize as a "bruise." The presence or absence of bruising is often helpful to our visualization of who hit what in a crash. Most often though, it is the skeleton's structural damage that helps us to understand what happened to an occupant in a car crash.

After this chapter develops a useful understanding of the structure and vulnerability of bones, joints, ligaments, muscles and tendons, subsequent chapters will deal with crash injuries as they concern each of the major body segments, which we will consider to be the:

- **Extremities**
    - lower extremities (including the hip joint and pelvis)
    - upper extremities (including the shoulder joint)
- **Chest** (thorax) and its contents
- **Abdomen** and its contents
- **Head and Face** and their contents (i.e., including brain injuries)
- **Spine** and its contents (including vertebrae, sacrum, coccyx and spinal cord)

THE SKELETON

We shall approach the skeleton from a non-classical anatomic viewpoint, that of an axially loaded series of columns, as shown in figure 18. There we placed the head of a 150 lb man, weighing about 9.1 pounds (skin, stuffing and all), onto the vertebral column (figure 18a). The shovel-shaped fused bones of the sacrum and coccyx were then hooked into the pelvic bones (figure 18b). Lastly, we engaged the socket joints (acetabulae) of the pelvis onto the ball portions of the hip joint, at the upper end of the lower extremity columns, thus assembling the entire weight bearing portion of the skeleton (figure 18c).

It certainly looks like something is missing from this skeleton, say, ribs, breast bone (sternum) and upper extremities. But we said this is the weight bearing (axially loaded) skeleton, and neither the rib cage nor the upper limbs are weight bearing, are they?

We will now form a full skeleton by attaching twelve pairs of ribs and the upper limbs. Note that ribs attach at notches in their respectively numbered thoracic vertebrae (see figure 19a), at the upper back portion of the body of the vertebra and also at a second facet on the transverse process of the same vertebra. We will also attach the upper ten of the twelve pairs of ribs to the sternum, by means of cartilaginous extensions. Four ribs (2 pairs) only attach in the back, to vertebrae. Anteriorly, (in the front) these ribs float free of bony attachments (see figure 19b).

Next we will hang the upper limbs to . . . to . . . to where? My goodness! The upper limbs really don't appear to attach to anything! They don't plug into a true socket, as the lower limbs did into the hip sockets. And where do the shoulder blades attach?

On close inspection, we do find a sort of tenuous connection to the rest of the skeleton; there is a pair of horizontal bones, the collar bones (clavicles), in the upper (superior) front (anterior) aspect of the upper breast bone (the manubrium).

So the collarbones attach to the chest, at the upper sides of the breast bone. It sure is a small attachment for an appendage the size of the upper extremity; it is less than an inch of tissue. Curiously, it is a joint quite similar to the knee and jaw joints in that a cartilaginous disc is interposed between the bones, and a fibrous capsule then envelopes the joint, extending from bone to bone. A similar joint, cartilage meniscus and all, exists at the opposite end of the collar bone, at the articulation with the acromion, a bony extension of the scapula. If we wish to exercise a teleological option, we may presume that the sternoclavicular and acromioclavicular joints are often loaded with many pounds per square inch, since where else the body has interposed such cartilagious discs into a joint, such joints have been relatively highly loaded.

This diminutive sterno-clavicular joint, it turns out, is the only hard connection of the upper limb to the rest of the skeleton.

While it is true that the shoulder blade (scapula) attaches to the clavicle and the upper arm bone (humerus) with several good-sized ligaments — composed of course of fibrous bands of connective tissue, preponderately collagen — only the collar bones connect directly to the rest of the skeleton. The shoulder blades (scapulae) attach to the skeleton only by muscles. These muscles are arranged to nearly completely encircle the shoulder joint, which makes for an extraordinarily mobile joint — witness how you can raise and lower your shoulders and arms and how you can also slide them forward and rearward while rotating them too. The large and relatively numerous muscles that fasten the shoulder to the trunk make for a good shock absorbing system as well as for a quite mobile joint, albeit a joint that is just barely attached to the rest of the skeleton.

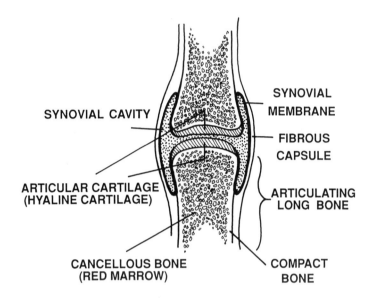

SYNOVIAL CAVITY

SYNOVIAL MEMBRANE

FIBROUS CAPSULE

ARTICULATING LONG BONE

ARTICULAR CARTILAGE (HYALINE CARTILAGE)

CANCELLOUS BONE (RED MARROW)

COMPACT BONE

Figure 20
THE SYNOVIAL JOINT

This is our usual joint; the type of joint we identify with our fingers and toes. It occurs wherever long bones articulate, not only in our fingers and toes, but also in our hands and feet, our elbows and knees and our shoulders and hips.

The joint surfaces that contact each other are faced with a distinct and remarkably smooth material, called hyaline (that means "glassy") cartilage. They are lubricated by a film of locally produced and secreted synovial fluid that has mechanical properties quite similar to petroleum lubricants.

If the smooth articulating surfaces are made rough or irregular, as in fractures through the articulating surfaces (and with certain diseases), they rapidly wear, producing a characteristic pathologic process that we term "osteo-arthritis," resulting in a painful, progressive restriction of joint motion.

We've now managed to assemble an entire skeleton (figure 19c). While we also could attach some 220 muscles to the skeleton from what are their tendinous origins and insertions, let us rather concentrate on how muscles attach to each other and to bones, and how bones connect to other bones (i.e., joints). We need to know about such things before we understand how we do violence to them.

Muscles and Tendons

Muscles are invested by a sheet of fibrous connective tissue (fascia), which lines body walls and extremities, separating some muscles and grouping other muscles into functional units.

Various fascial layers extend beyond muscles, attaching them to bone or to another muscle as a sheet of connective tissue (called an aponeurosis), or to the periosteum (outer layer of bones) by a cord-like extension of fascia termed a "tendon."

Tendons and aponeuroses can themselves be cut or torn in a crash or they can tear loose from either bone or muscle, often taking with them a piece of the bone at their attachment point (viz., an "avulsion fracture").

Joints

The regions where bones articulate with each other are called "joints." They are quite variable and often also quite complex, but they may be divided into three large categories:

fibrous joints, which have no joint cavity and therefore are almost without movement; they are simply bones held fast to each other by fibrous, largely collagenous, connective tissue. Examples include the way the flat bones of the skull and breast bones are joined.

cartilaginous joints, which also have no joint cavity and very little movement. Bone is joined to bone by cartilage, a very dense connective tissue different from other connective tissue by, among other things, absence of blood vessels or nerves. Examples include the joint between ribs and the breast bone and between the bodies of vertebrae, where the cartilage is a variant called "fibrocartilage."

synovial joints. These are the joints most people think of when they bother to think at all about the joints between articulating bones. These synovial joints have a space between the bones, called (of course) the synovial joint cavity.

Where the bones touch each other they are lined with hyaline cartilage, a slick, smooth, glassy, load-distributing surface. Hyaline cartilage is without any of its own blood vessels, which makes it *almost* devoid therefore of any ability to heal itself when damaged.

A two layered sleeve encloses the joint, the inner layer secreting a complex fluid which actually lubricates the joint, and a fibrous outer layer connecting bone to bone, selectively thickened in certain area into fibrous connective tissue bands called ligaments. All this can be seen in figure 20.

Ligaments

Ligaments function both as strength members, attaching bone to bone as well as stabilizing the joint and limiting its range of motion. Ligaments may be within the joint itself, as in the cruciate ligaments of the knee joint, although the usual ligament may be considered to be either external to or part of the joint capsule.

Tears of a ligament are technically termed a **sprain** and should not be used interchangeably with or confused with the term **strain**, the latter being a tear of a musculotendinous unit[6]. (There is an exception to that: repeated stretching of a ligament, in the absence of a tear, is called a "ligamentous strain.") But let me repeat and emphasize that a tear of the connective tissue connecting bone-to-bone, a ligament, is called a **sprain**; a tear of muscle fibers and/or their tendon fibers is properly termed a **strain**. Because they describe quite different damage, different mechanisms of injury, possibly different treatment and possibly different disability consequences, *they should not be used interchangeably*.

A CLOSER LOOK AT BONES

Depending on how they are counted, there are between 200 and 206 bones in the average adult skeleton, (the numbers vary because anatomists do not always agree with each other as to what is a what), but most anatomists do agree that bones can be classified by shape, recognizing four major types and four other types:

long bones—are dense tubes, longer then they are wide. They grow spongy inside and are covered by smooth cartilage at each end;
short bones—are found only in the wrist and foot. They are about cuboidal in

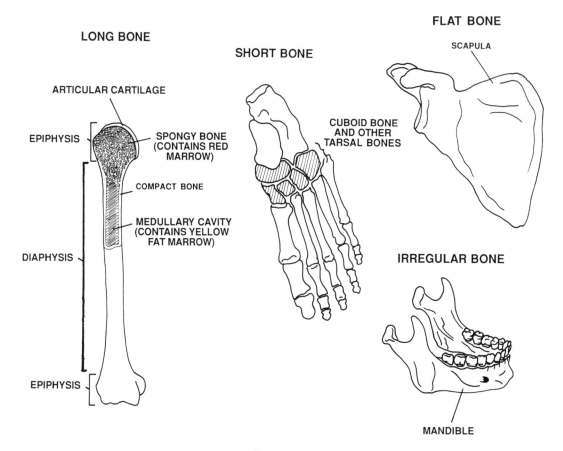

Figure 21
THE FOUR MOST COMMON TYPES OF BONES

Long bones' architecture is of particular note because the bulbous ends of the bones (the epiphysis at each end of a long bone) contain a spongy, trabeculated bony core, similar to a solid open foam in both its form and in its ability to absorb energy when deformed.

The hollow tube of the shaft (diaphysis) of the long bones is a shape well designed to be particularly strong in compression for its weight, so it is not surprising to find such tubes in all four of our limbs, reminding us again that we are derived from four-legged ancestors.

Short bones exist in the wrist and the foot, serving well to produce limited multi-directional motion under load.

Flat bones, as in the scapula, sternum and skull, have great stiffness and strength for their weight, in both torsion and bending. The same design is utilized for these same virtues in modern construction panels in which a stiff foam is sandwiched between two compact outer layers.

Irregular bones, such as the jaw and facial bones, are just that, irregular bones, some with symmetry and some without.

Bones such as vertebrae have some features common to more than one bony type, the vertebral bodies being similar to long bones and the vertebral arches being similar to irregular bones. That some bones do not fit well our classification should serve as reminder that it is we who are trying to force them into our classification; I doubt that bones care much how well they fit our typification.

shape, although they may have more than four surfaces;

flat bones—two plates of dense compact bone with a middle layer of spongy bone, stuffed with marrow, as in the skull;

irregular bones—such as in the face and vertebrae,

as well as pneumatic, accessory, sesamoid and heterotopic bones, these last four types not being considered here.

See figure 21 for the appearance of the four most common types of bones.

With this very basic description of bones, joints, ligaments, tendons and muscle now beneath our belts, we will now turn to musculoskeletal injuries.

HOW TO WREAK MUSCULOSKELETAL HAVOC

There are two ways that force can be applied to the body and cause injuries: first by the *direct* application of force, such as hitting someone on a scapula with a hammer and thereby breaking it. Second, by *indirect* application of force, by transmitted force, as when we fall on the outstretched open pronated hand, transmitting the force from wrist bones (carpi) to the distal forearm bones — primarily to the radius — and then to the humerus, scapula and clavicle. Such falls may fracture the wrist, forearm, or collar bone by force transmitted along the chain of connected bones.

With regard to the scapula, by the way, to my knowledge it can *only* be broken by a direct blow and therefore a fractured scapula tells us much, and this is true of other flat bones and some irregular bones too.

What a broken flat bone tells us is this: if it is broken, it was probably struck directly, where it is broken.

In addition, because the scapula is such a large, strong bone, its fracture tells us that a large amount of force was involved and that therefore we'd better look for other injuries nearby, especially to the lung, chest wall, shoulder joint and the major blood vessels, all nearby and all on the same side as the fractured scapula[8].

Wrecking Bones

We've discussed fractures briefly, noting that they are caused largely by four directions of forces: tension, torsion, compression and shear. (Bending, you may recall, is tension on one side of the bone and compression on the opposite side.)

More commonly in trauma, fractures occur from combinations of these forces, and the directions of the damage-causing stresses may be interpreted from the damage they rendered unto bone, including such other loading characteristics as its relative magnitude and/or the rate of loading.

Some Different Fractures

The terminology of fractures is not obscure. Most terms, if not self evident, are easily clarified by a medical dictionary. The following terms are probably well known to all readers, but will be used frequently in the following chapters and are presented here for convenience. A large number of terms are not given that are specific for childrens' fracture terminology, joint fracture classification and so forth. Reference[10] in the next chapter is the most convenient fracture classification source handbook that I have found.

- **Complicated Fracture:** involves injury to nerves, blood vessels or proximate organs, as with a fractured rib perforating the lung beneath the rib.
- **Comminuted Fracture:** has more than two significant fragments.
- **Crush Fracture:** requires crush of the trabeculae of cancellous bone.
- **"Open" or "Compound" Fracture:** the fracture site is associated with an open wound connecting to "outside." The wound can be from within, from bone fragments piercing outward, or from an external object piercing the skin.
- **Displaced Fracture:** the fracture fragments are not in anatomic position.

Wrecking Joints

While we note that joints are classifiable into: 1) immovable joints, 2) slightly movable joints, and 3) freely movable joints, (viz., synarthroses, amphiarthroses and diarthroses, respectively), we will here concern ourselves only with the freely movable joints because their injuries require the most treatment and because their injuries cause the greatest disabilities of the various joint injuries. However, we should appreciate that when they are injured, the less movable joints entail fracture or fracture-dislocations, since their very immobility renders them less able to dissipate energy.

Earlier in this chapter, when we classified joints, we called the freely movable joints "synovial joints," indicating thereby that these movable joints were lined with a lubricant-producing joint capsule, (the synovium), and that the surfaces bearing against each other were formed of hyaline cartilage, which is slick, smooth and bloodless.

Joint injuries are, after simple bruises, the second most common type of trauma seen in clinical practice and are second only to severe fractures for the number of days of disability they produce[9].

Synovial joint injuries are divisible into:

- **disruptions of motion** or
- **disruptions of stability**.

Joint motion disruption can occur with or without changes in stability, as in fragments of a knee meniscus "locking" the joint, or with tearing of an internal ligament, such as the anterior or posterior cruciate ligament.

Joint stability disruption is most commonly caused by torn external ligaments secondary to a joint being forced beyond its normal range of motion. The joint is stressed in tension, causing the bony components to fail (fracture) and/or the fibrous capsule and ligaments to fail (tear), in tension. **The causative force in joint (tension) failure usually is an indirect force, a transmitted stress**[10].

PATTERNS OF SKELETAL CRASH INJURIES

Since 1971, when the first Abbreviated Injury Scale (AIS) was published under the joint sponsorship of the American Medical Association and the American Association for Automotive Medicine, almost all crash injury publications have reported injuries in terms of the Abbreviated Injury Scale, i.e., AIS 1-6. Under this system, injuries "equivalent" in terms primarily of "threat-to-life" bear the same number (from 1 to 6), with increasingly higher numbers inferring greater threat to life. This system, we will later find, will necessarily equate say, a below-the-knee amputation with say, a full thickness perforation of the anus. Both of these injuries would rate a 3, which is to say that they are both termed as "serious" in the scale. Clearly, the disability consequences of a below-the-knee amputation and a rectal tear are enormously different, although their threat-to-life consequences emergently may well have been equal, or "serious."

While this reporting system may be of real need or convenience to some — such as some statisticians — and may serve to distract or mislead others — such as other statisticians, for purposes of defining patterns of skeletal injuries in crash we will necessarily have to go back to pre-1971 reports and more recent clinical publications.

The various injury scales, mainly the AIS, used in automotive journals since 1971 have, with only few exceptions, replaced the reporting of specific injuries and therefore largely corrupted the literature for anyone interested in anything more detailed than injury scale numbers.

This book will later have a small chapter on injury scales and what they mean in terms of their obfuscation of the evaluation of success or failure of vehicle modifications. For now we will look at some musculo-skeletal crash injury epidemiology.

As a start we have a 1979 study from Denmark reported in terms of both actual data and the Abbreviated Injury Scale[11]. The injuries are defined as "bone and joint" injuries that happened to 200 car occupants injured and brought to the emergency room at Odense University Hospital in Odense, Denmark, from 1972 to 1979. The data in table 5 of that report has been recalculated from that report and is presented here in our table 3:

TABLE 3 (from ref.[11])

Region of Skeleton	Bone or Joint Injury (% of total)
Head (includes face)	20%
Spine (includes pelvis)	11.5%
Chest (ribs and sternum)	18.5%
Upper extremities	31.5%
Lower extremities	18.5%
	100.0%

Remember, this was just the distribution of bone and joint injuries in injured occupant survivors of automotive crashes. What I found so interesting about this study was that bony injuries to the arms was clearly more common than injury to any other region. Let's look at another study to see what it says.

From a 1956 study of the distribution of fractures among 661 hospitalized U.S. motorist casualties[12] we derived table 4:

TABLE 4 (from ref[12])

Region of Skeleton	Bone or Joint Injury (fracture %)
Head (includes face)	26%
Spine (includes pelvis)	15%
Chest (ribs and sternum)	21%
All extremities	38%
	100%

Lastly, we'll look at a study reported in 1988 by radiologists, who thankfully have no apparent reason to report injuries in terms of trauma scales and simply let it all hang out. Their study was of the injuries to 250 unrestrained drivers and 250 unrestrained passengers involved in frontal collisions while traveling 35 mph or greater, without ejections, treated at the trauma center at the Allegheny General Hospital in 1985[13]. Please note that the body regions here included soft tissue injuries to the head and chest.

TABLE 5 (from ref[13])

Region of Skeleton	Bone or Joint Injury (% of total)		
	driver	passenger	both
Head (including face)	11.8%	21.5%	16.7%
Spine (including pelvis)	16.9%	17.6%	17.3%
Chest (ribs and sternum)	10.3%	10.9%	10.6%
Upper extremities	22.1%	21.3%	21.7%
Lower extremities	39.9%	28.7%	33.8%
	100.0%	100.0%	100.1%

It is noteworthy that there were about 50 percent more driver skeletal injuries than there were passenger skeletal injuries. The distribution of skeletal injuries was nearly identical between them, except that drivers sustained a third more lower limb bony injuries than the passengers, and the passengers incurred nearly twice the incidence of skull and facial fractures. Do remember that these were unrestrained occupants of frontal impacts, and that we can still expect about 50 percent of car crash occupants currently to remain unrestrained, despite our laws and educational programs.

That also means that about 50 percent of the car occupants involved in crashes will be or are currently restrained.

So before leaving the topic, we will put together another simple table, this time of *restrained* frontal car crash occupants who sustained at least one injury of AIS 2 or greater (that is, a "moderate" injury or greater), as reported by Dalmotas in 1980[14]. Remember these are not just skeletal injuries; these are all injuries sustained and reported as "moderate" or worse. Because the body regions used in ref.[14] do not correspond to those reported in the tables above, the regional distribution will be less than 100 percent. (The difference appears to be largely due to the omission of spine injuries from table 6.) And again, this table has been recalculated by me from data given in ref.[14].

TABLE 6 (from ref.[14])

Body Region	**Percent AIS 2 or Greater** (driver + front passenger)
Head/face (includes brain)	29.7%
Chest (includes shoulder)	22.5%
Abdomen (includes pelvis)	13.2%
Upper extremities (less shoulder)	12.6%
Lower extremities (less pelvis)	17.8%
	95.8%

These tables (3 to 6) have a bit to say to us:

1) Whether the measure of injury is skeletal damage or all "moderate" or greater injuries, **the extremities are the most commonly injured regions.** As expected, this is true whether or not the occupant is restrained, because the extremities themselves never are restrained, are they?

2) Again, whether restrained or not and whether the injuries are limited to bony damage only — or bony and soft tissues too — **the head (including the face) is the second most commonly injured region.** The head, like the extremities, also is not

restrained, except in those restraints that include air bags as a supplemental part of the system.

3) Studies seem to vary substantially in whether or not the lower or the upper extremities have the higher incidence of skeletal injuries. The Danish study[11] suggests that upper extremity bone and joint crash injuries are nearly twice as common as lower extremity; the Pittsburgh study[13] found the reverse to be true, that lower extremity injuries were more than 50 percent more common than upper extremity injuries, but the Pittsburgh study was limited to relatively high energy frontal crashes and the Danish study was not so limited.

4) The Pittsburgh study also showed a marked difference between injury patterns of driver and right front occupant, the unrestrained right front occupants suffering nearly twice as many head injuries as did the drivers, and having a third less lower extremity injuries than did the drivers. Interestingly, the difference in lower limb injuries was attributable to the absence of ankle and foot injuries among the right front seat occupants. We'll address why this may be so in the next chapter, which is about crash injuries of the extremities.

SUMMARY

We early assembled a skeleton in order to get some idea of how our bones and joints are put together, then reviewed the various kinds of bones, joints and connective tissues associated with bones and joints, i.e., ligaments, joint capsules, tendons, cartilage and muscle.

We looked at how bones, joints and their associated tissues are injured — by direct or transmitted (indirect) forces — then functionally classified joint injuries as to whether they caused problems of joint motion or joint stability. We hardly classified fractures except as whether they were caused by an avulsion, tension, compression, torsion, shear or some combination thereof. We also did classify fractures as to whether the external investing tissues were open to the fracture site or closed to it, i.e., into "open" or "closed" fractures, noting that open fractures not only looked awful, they often had treatment and disability problems as awful as they looked.

Finally, we looked at the distribution of bone and joint injuries, noting that extremity injuries clearly were the most common crash injuries involving bones and joints, and, when combined, extremity injuries were in fact the most common crash injuries. Furthermore and importantly, current restraint systems don't seem to alter the incidence of extremity bone and joint injuries, possibly because neither upper nor lower limbs are restrained in any of our current restraint systems.

BIBLIOGRAPHY

1. Tortora, G.J. and N.P. Anagnostakos: *Principles of Anatomy.* 5th Ed., Harper & Row, New York, 1987.
(This is a useful text, written for nurses' training and for paramedical specialties, such as medical and laboratory technicians. The authors contend that their text assumes the reader has had no prior study of the human body.)

2. Moore, K.L.: *Clinically Oriented Anatomy.* 2nd Ed., Williams & Wilkins, Baltimore, 1985.
(This is for first year anatomy students, but it is not a "core" anatomy text, rather it is a clinically oriented supplement to an anatomy text, providing some clinical insight, surface anatomy, radiology and other information not generally available in classical anatomy texts.)

3. Gardner, E., Gray, D.J., and R. O'Rahilly: *Anatomy.* 4th Ed., W.B. Saunders Co., Philadelphia, 1975.
(This is a typical core anatomy text for medical students. There are many other equivalent texts that should perhaps be selected on the basis of personal preference or readability to you, the reader. Visit your local medical school bookstore.)

4. Netter, F.H.: *Atlas of Human Anatomy.* Ciba-Geigy Corp., West Caldwell, N.J., 1989.
(This is certainly the best single anatomy atlas I have known, by the late master medical illustrator, Frank H. Netter, M.D.)

5. Gozna, E.R., Harrington, I.J. and D.C. Evans: *Biomechanics of Musculoskeletal Injury.* Williams & Wilkins, Baltimore p. 2, 1982.

6. Ogilvie-Harris, D.J. and G.J. Lloyd: *Personal Injury.* Canada Law Book, Inc., Toronto p. 43, 1986.

7. Clayman, C.B.: *AMA Encyclopedia of Medicine.* Random House, New York, 1989.

8. Thompson, D.A., Flynn, T.C., Miller, P.W. and R.P. Fischer: The significance of scapular fractures. *J Trauma 25*:10, p. 974-977, 1985.

9. Nahum, A.M. and J. Melvin (Eds.): *The Biomechanics of Trauma.* Appleton-Century-Crofts, Norwalk p. 375, 1985.

10. Salter, R.B.: *Textbook of Disorders and Injuries of the Musculoskeletal System.* 2nd Ed., Williams & Wilkins, Baltimore p. 418-419, 1983.

11. Jorgensen, J., Kruse, T., Somers, R.L. and R. Weeth: Description of 3225

victims of road-traffic-accident trauma according to type of accident, severity of unjury, and nature of lesions sustained. *IVth International IRCOBI Conference on the Biomechanics of Trauma*, 1979. (Calculated from data in Table 5, p. 20).

12. Kulowski, J.: *Crash Injuries.* Charles C Thomas, Springfield p. 301, fig. 154, 1960.

13. Daffner, R.H., Deeb, Z.L., Lupetin, A.R. and W.E. Rothfus: Patterns of high-speed impact injuries in motor vehicle occupants. *J Trauma 28*:4, p. 498-501, 1988.

14. Dalmotas, D.J.: Mechanisms of injury to vehicle occupants restrained by three-point seat belts. *SAE* paper 801311, 1980.

CHAPTER 5

CRASH INJURIES OF THE EXTREMITIES

GENERAL

In the volumes written about crash injuries, not much has been devoted to the extremities. Of what little has been written about extremity injuries, almost all of it is concerned with the lower extremities.

The fact is, I've not found a single publication, not a single technical journal article wholly devoted to crash injuries of the upper extremities. There are occasional clinical case reports and the like for relatively "oddball" events, such as the possible relationship between vehicular crash and, say, carpal tunnel syndrome[1]. And upper extremity injuries are often reported as part of regional tolerance and regional injury distribution, but I've yet to see a single article solely concerned with the mechanics of upper extremity impact injury, the evaluation of upper extremity vehicle crash injury impairments, or consideration of possible mechanisms to prevent such injuries.

I do not know why both of the extremities are so neglected, because, as we saw in the previous chapter in each of four quite different studies, *the extremities are the most frequently injured regions of the bony skeleton or of the entire body, however you choose to look at it.*

"Injuries cause impairments; impairments cause disabilities."[2] The cost to society of extremity injuries and their resultant impairments and disabilities is now well documented as the sum of its costs: administrative, medical treatment, rehabilitation, workmens' compensation, social security and loss of income[3]. According to ref. [3], for example, the cost of an open fracture of the humerus (upper arm) with subsequent impairment has a societal cost about a third of that of a cervical fracture with complete quadriplegia; that of a simple closed fracture of a hip joint with residual functional impairment costs society about two-thirds as much as a cervical fracture with quadriplegia!

Clearly, we're not neglecting the study of common extremity injuries because they are not costly to society.

Are we not writing much about upper extremity injuries because we can do so little about them? That is, we don't study them much because we don't tie them down with restraints? I doubt that; we don't directly restrain the head either, but I would guess that we've devoted more study to head injuries than to any other crash injury.

In short, I have no idea why upper extremity injuries with their resultant disabilities and their extraordinary long term costs have not been more vigorously studied, nor why lower extremity injuries with even greater disability potential have not had more vigorous crashworthiness consideration, more vigorous interest in their prevention.

Am I simply not aware of what has been written? It certainly is possible, but I do doubt it.

McElhaney, Roberts and Hilyard's "Handbook of Human Tolerance" discusses lower limb injuries but does not address upper limb injuries as such; Nahum and Melvin's "The Biomechanics of Trauma" does cover the biomechanics and clinical aspects of extremity injuries but does not touch the causality of crash injuries of upper and lower extremities; Melvin and Weber's recent fine "Review of Biomechanical Impact Response and Injury in the Automotive Environment" sponsored by NHTSA, has a chapter on the lower extremities but has nothing at all about upper extremities; the SAE has published a special volume on "Biomechanics and Medical Aspects of Lower Limb Injuries," but the SAE has not published anything about the upper limbs; finally, SAE J885 (1986), "Human Tolerance to Impact Conditions as Related to Motor Vehicle Design" has in it nothing at all about foot/ankle injuries, although they represent a quarter of all lower limb crash injuries[4], and has nothing at all to say about upper extremity crash injuries, which represent about 1 out of every 5 or 6 crash injuries.

My goodness, even J.A. Pike's "Automotive Safety: Anatomy, Injury, Testing and Regulation," published by the SAE in 1990, has nothing to say about our upper limbs; it doesn't even list the upper extremities under the chapter heading of "Anatomy and Injury!" Upper extremities, I guess, simply are not part of "automotive safety."

So maybe it is simply that hardly anyone — and this includes the National Highway Traffic Safety Administration for at least these past twenty-five years — hardly anyone seems to care that upper extremity crash injuries can and do cause devastating and costly disabilities, that upper and lower extremity injuries together are *the* most common crash injuries and, together, extremity injuries surely are *the* most common cause of permanent impairment and disability resulting from motor vehicle accidents.

Or maybe it is that automotive safety is regulation-driven, all auto manufacturers' statements to the contrary notwithstanding. Without specified safety requirements and the clout to compel compliance with such safety requirements, automotive manufacturers as a group just should not by and of themselves be expected to advance automotive safety state-of-the-art.

Or maybe it is that automotive safety regulations are consumer lobby-driven, all National Highway Traffic Safety Administration statements to the contrary notwithstanding. Unless consumer organizations themselves study and understand what the problems are — and then lobby to have NHTSA do something about the problems — NHTSA may not by and of itself advance the automotive safety state-of-the-art, (although it should be expected to do so).

Are we expecting too much when we expect that *someone* out there, federal or manufacturer, has some responsibility to identify the important traffic accident causes of both death and disability, and then has some responsibility to do something about curable causes of both death and disability?

Somebody? Anybody, out there?

CRASH INJURIES OF THE LOWER EXTREMITIES

Here's a general rule that I find useful for preponderantly *frontal collisions*: **all lower limb injuries below the knee are generally due to toe pan, floor pan and firewall intrusion, and only rarely to interaction with the driver's pedals. All knee, thigh and hip injuries are due to contact with the dash or steering column.**

For preponderantly *lateral collisions,* **as above, plus: all lower limb injuries on the same-side-occupants' same side as the collision, including injuries to the pelvis, may be additionally due to lateral intrusion of the same-side door and/or of the same-side floor pan. Injuries to the same-side-occupant that occur on the side opposite the collision may be additionally due to collision with opposite-side occupants.**

The Distribution of Lower Limb Injuries

By now we should be aware that in comparing injury incidence from one study to another there will be differences in both what constitutes an injury sufficient for inclusion in any one study and what is included within a body region (e.g., is an intra-articular fracture through a femoral condyle considered "thigh" or considered "knee?"). With such limitations in mind, let us compare four different studies to determine the distribution of lower limb injuries:

TABLE 7

The Distribution of Lower Limb Injuries

Region	% of Lower Limb Injuries				Study [reference]
Pelvis/hip	16.0 [6]	13.3 [4]	11.1 [7]	22.8 [5]	
Thigh	18	11.5	36.5	27.9	
Knee	17.5	26.3	13.2	8.8	
Leg	21	30.3	18.7	15.0	
Foot/ankle	27.5	18.5	24.6	25.6	

Admittedly, I've mixed a few apples and oranges here, but of the five regions of the lower limb, the foot/ankle seems to be consistently one of every four or five injuries.

Reference[4] seems most disparate from the other studies [5] [6] [7] and perhaps this is best explained by the fact that only in reference[4] is the data from frontal, side and rear accidents; in the other three studies [5] [6] [7] the data was filtered to deal only with frontal impacts.

The following specific fractures and fracture mechanisms will read about as smoothly as — and have all the innate charm of — an encyclopedia, a modest version of which it may be. If you don't have specific interest in a specific injury mechanism, you can save the reading of some or all of these injury mechanism sections until you do have such need. Or you may just want to scan them now to know their contents, for possible future needs and use. You choose.

Now let's have a closer look at the five anatomic regions of the lower extremity, starting with injuries at the bottom, at the feet, and working our way upwards to the bony pelvis (but not the pelvic contents).

We will deal with the foot and ankle together, as if they were a single unit, partly because they operate together as a complex single functional unit and partly because that is the way that foot and ankle injuries are usually reported in both clinical and crash injury literature.

The Foot and Ankle

Accident injury surveys claim that 20 to 30 percent of lower limb injuries involve

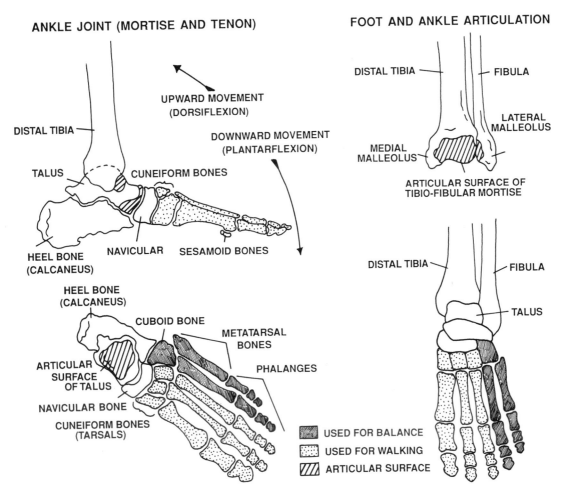

ANKLE JOINT (MORTISE AND TENON)

UPWARD MOVEMENT
(DORSIFLEXION)

DOWNWARD MOVEMENT
(PLANTARFLEXION)

DISTAL TIBIA

TALUS   CUNEIFORM BONES

HEEL BONE
(CALCANEUS)

NAVICULAR   SESAMOID BONES

HEEL BONE
(CALCANEUS)

CUBOID BONE

METATARSAL
BONES

ARTICULAR
SURFACE
OF TALUS

PHALANGES

NAVICULAR BONE

CUNEIFORM BONES
(TARSALS)

FOOT AND ANKLE ARTICULATION

DISTAL TIBIA   FIBULA

LATERAL
MALLEOLUS

MEDIAL
MALLEOLUS

ARTICULAR SURFACE OF
TIBIO-FIBULAR MORTISE

DISTAL TIBIA   FIBULA

TALUS

USED FOR BALANCE
USED FOR WALKING
ARTICULAR SURFACE

Figure 22
THE FOOT AND THE ANKLE ARTICULATIONS

Our feet and our hands are analogous. The differences between our hands and feet relate to our hands retaining flexibility and mobility while our feet are distinctly set up for weight bearing and balance.

The lateral (outer) margins of our feet contribute to balance while the three innermost toes and the bones that connect with them (metatarsals and tarsal bones) lead to the heel and to the *tenon* of the ankle joint, the talus, and thus are primarily load bearing or load transmitting bones.

The two bony projections that most of us think of as "ankle" are termed "malleoli" or, as the venerable Greek anatomists somehow saw it, as the diminutive form of a hammer. The ankle joint is formed by the tibia, which transmits nearly all of the body's weight, — and its extension, which forms the medial malleolus — and the fibula, which scarcely transmits any vertical load at all — and its extension, the lateral malleolus — which stabilizes the joint. Together, the distal tibia and fibula form the *mortise* of the ankle joint, and are held together as a mortise and tenon joint by numerous ligaments, some of which are shown in figures 23 and 25.

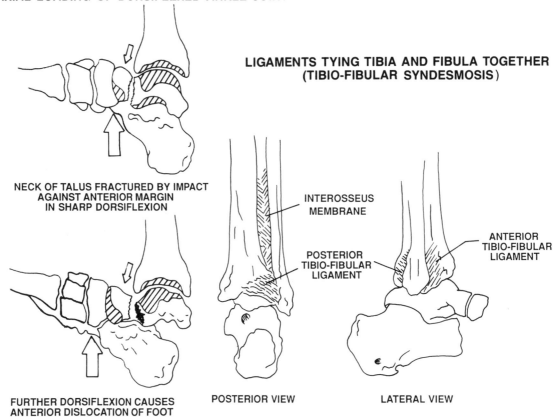

FRACTURE OF TALUS RESULTING FROM AXIAL LOADING OF DORSIFLEXED ANKLE JOINT

NECK OF TALUS FRACTURED BY IMPACT AGAINST ANTERIOR MARGIN IN SHARP DORSIFLEXION

FURTHER DORSIFLEXION CAUSES ANTERIOR DISLOCATION OF FOOT

LIGAMENTS TYING TIBIA AND FIBULA TOGETHER (TIBIO-FIBULAR SYNDESMOSIS)

INTEROSSEUS MEMBRANE

POSTERIOR TIBIO-FIBULAR LIGAMENT

ANTERIOR TIBIO-FIBULAR LIGAMENT

POSTERIOR VIEW

LATERAL VIEW

Figure 23
TALAR FRACTURE DISLOCATION AND THE TIBIO-FIBULAR SYNDESMOSIS

These illustrations are both concerned with axial loading of the mortise and tenon joint of the ankle. (Figure 24 will show how these loads result from car crashes and figure 25 will show the mechanism of common bi- and tri-malleolar fractures.)

Forced dorsiflexion at the ankle joint when combined with modest axial loading may cause talar fracture, as shown above. When dorsiflexion is further forced, talar fracture will procede to dislocation, putting in jeopardy the posterior tibial nerve, artery and vein, as well as survival of the foot itself.

The other views of the ankle show ligaments that hold together the bones of the ankle mortise. Forced axial loading at the ankle joint combined with any other motion at the joint (except for the previously discussed dorsiflexion) may rupture or tear these ligaments. When torn, these ligaments then allow for some separation of the two sides of the ankle mortise, and therefore allow for play or looseness within the mortise and tenon joint of the ankle.

A loose or wobbly joint will rapidly wear. We term such rapid and excessive joint wear as "osteoarthritis" or "degenerative joint disease." No matter what we call it, it means that such joints quickly become painful and quickly lose flexibility. A painful, immobile joint is, in effect, no joint at all.

You may want to remember that there are two general indications for joint surgery: to restore mobility and/or to stop pain.

the foot and ankle, which in turn puts foot and ankle injuries at about 5 to 10 percent of all moderate or serious crash injuries[4] [5].

The foot is comprised of 26 bones, not counting accessory and sesamoid bones, the latter groups (except for the knee cap) having almost no clinical significance whatever.

The foot articulates with the mortise formed by the distal tibia and fibula (medial and lateral malleoli) by means of the talus, an irregular bone that rests on the heel bone (calcaneus). The distal tibia and fibula, with the upper articulating surface of the talus, form the hinge joint we call the ankle. See figure 22. When we call the ankle a hinge joint we mean that the attached foot can only move upwards (dorsiflex) and downwards (plantarflex).

Functionally, the foot should be divided into the first 3 toes — and their metatarsals, three cuneiforms and the navicular bone behind them — all of which are concerned with *walking and running*. The lateral fourth and fifth toes with their metatarsals and the cuboid bone behind (proximal to) them are all concerned with *balance*.

Our entire weight is transmitted through the ankle joint — the distal tibia carrying nearly all of our weight — to the foot, where our weight is borne by the heel (calcaneus) and distal first 3 metatarsal bones, especially the ball of the great toe.

(A couple of small sesamoid bones generally are slipped into the joint capsule just beneath the ball of the first toe "knuckle." But sesamoids are, like the knee cap, just bony nodules faced with articular cartilage that form inside of tendons at major wear points.)

As we walk our weight transfers from heel to first 3 toe knuckles, from heel to first 3 toe knuckles. Most of the foot fractures due to crash that I have seen involve the foot's lateral aspects (4th and 5th metatarsals and the cuboid bone) and have been associated with buckling of the floor pan and/or toe pan. The base of the fifth metatarsal is the site of *the* most common, albeit relatively trivial, foot fracture.

Crash injuries of the foot can be the cause of significant impairment or disability if they involve amputation or the loss of the arches of the foot or loss of mobility at *any* of the foot's many joints.

Fracture dislocation of *the talus* is a severe injury seen in both motorcycle and car accidents. It appears to result from axial loading of the fully dorsiflexed ankle joint. See figure 23. The talus fractures at its neck, in the coronal plane, extruding the body of the talus posteriorly and medially, contacting and often compromising the posterior tibial nerve, artery and vein. Naturally, when nerve, artery and vein are all compromised, the foot itself is compromised.

At best, the talus has a tenuous blood supply. Fractures involving the neck of the

MECHANISMS OF FOOT AND ANKLE INJURIES

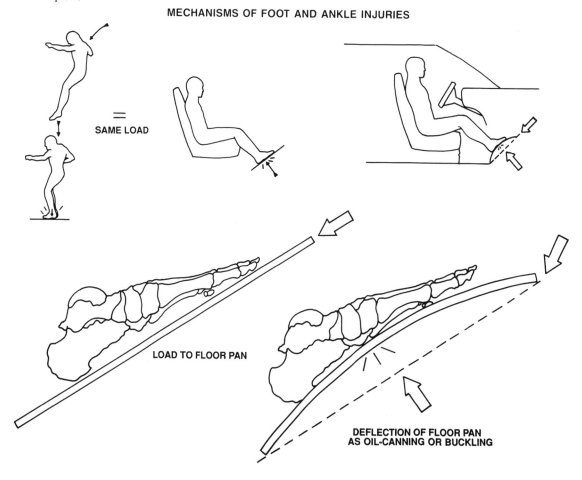

Figure 24
INJURIES OF THE FOOT, HEEL AND ANKLE, CAUSED BY
BUCKLING OF THE FRONT FLOOR PAN OR TOE PAN

The figures in the upper left illustrate that whether we fall down and strike the ground with a heel or whether the ground comes up and strikes a heel is identical in injury potential. If the magnitude of the forces involved are the same, the event is the same as far as the body is concerned, *because the resultant direction of force is identical.*

When the front or side of the thin metal plate that is a floor pan is struck and moved toward the center of the floor pan, as in frontal or lateral collisions, the floor pan may deflect or crumple, depending on how forcefully it was deformed and how far it was deflected. Modest movement will cause the floor pan to "oil can," which is a modest and impermanent deflection permitting the floor pan to elastically return to its original or near original position. Although oil canning is a modest metal movement, it involves force loadings that have great injury potential.

Either oil-canning or crumpling may slap the bottom of the foot with force sufficient to break one or more bones of the foot or ankle.

talus often have a late, frequent and unfortunate complication, that of "avascular necrosis," which is to say that the body of the talus literally dies for want of sufficient blood supply. This is a painful, significant impairment and, most often, a significant disability, as also is non-union of the talar fracture, another common complication related to its delicate blood supply.

The heel bone or *calcaneus* has four articulating surfaces; an anterior surface for the cuboid bone and three surfaces for the talus. The back portion of the heel is the attachment point (i.e., insertion) of the Achilles tendon, a very substantial tendon derived from the sheaths of the calf muscles. Because the calcaneus is made of cancellous bone, it is crushable. Because it is cancellous bone, it has a generous blood supply and therefore, as a rule, heels heal easily and rapidly.

It is the same load to the heel bone whether we fall from a height or if the ground somehow comes up and hits the bottom of the heel. The body does not distinguish between these events. When the floor pan buckles from early intrusion into the passenger compartment, it may "oil can," a term describing a thin flat metal plate's sudden deflection when a load is put upon the plate's margin. See figure 24. The floor pan literally slaps the bottom of the foot and the foot or ankle may be injured, as if we had fallen on the foot from a substantial height.

The most important ligaments of the ankle and foot, if we had to designate such, would surely be the ligaments that tie together the tibia and fibula (the interosseous membrane and the anterior and posterior tibio-fibular ligaments; see figure 23). These ligaments of the distal tibio-fibular joint together are referred to as the "tibio-fibular syndesmosis." (Of course, most of the ligaments of the foot and ankle have some importance and significant injury to any ligament can cause some impairment). But the tibio-fibular syndesmosis holds these two bones together as the mortise for the ankle joint's tenon, the talus. If the syndesmosis is torn, it is as if a wooden mortise and tenon joint were split; the joint will wobble badly and rapidly wear itself away even if the bones are still capable of transmitting force (weight) across the joint that remains.

There are many explanations and classifications of ankle joint fractures, but we will here use the explanation of Dr. R.B. Salter[8] because it is simple, current, and based upon the mechanics of the fractures. We will use the classification of Gozna and Harrington[9] for the same reasons. (It may be noted that almost all current concepts of the classification and mechanics of ankle injuries are to a large extent derived from J. Grant Bonnin's 1950 book *"Injuries to the Ankle"* published by Wm. Heinemann, London, an authoritative and clear exposition about that complex joint.)

(NOTE: Simple and low cost sources of general orthopedic fracture classifications

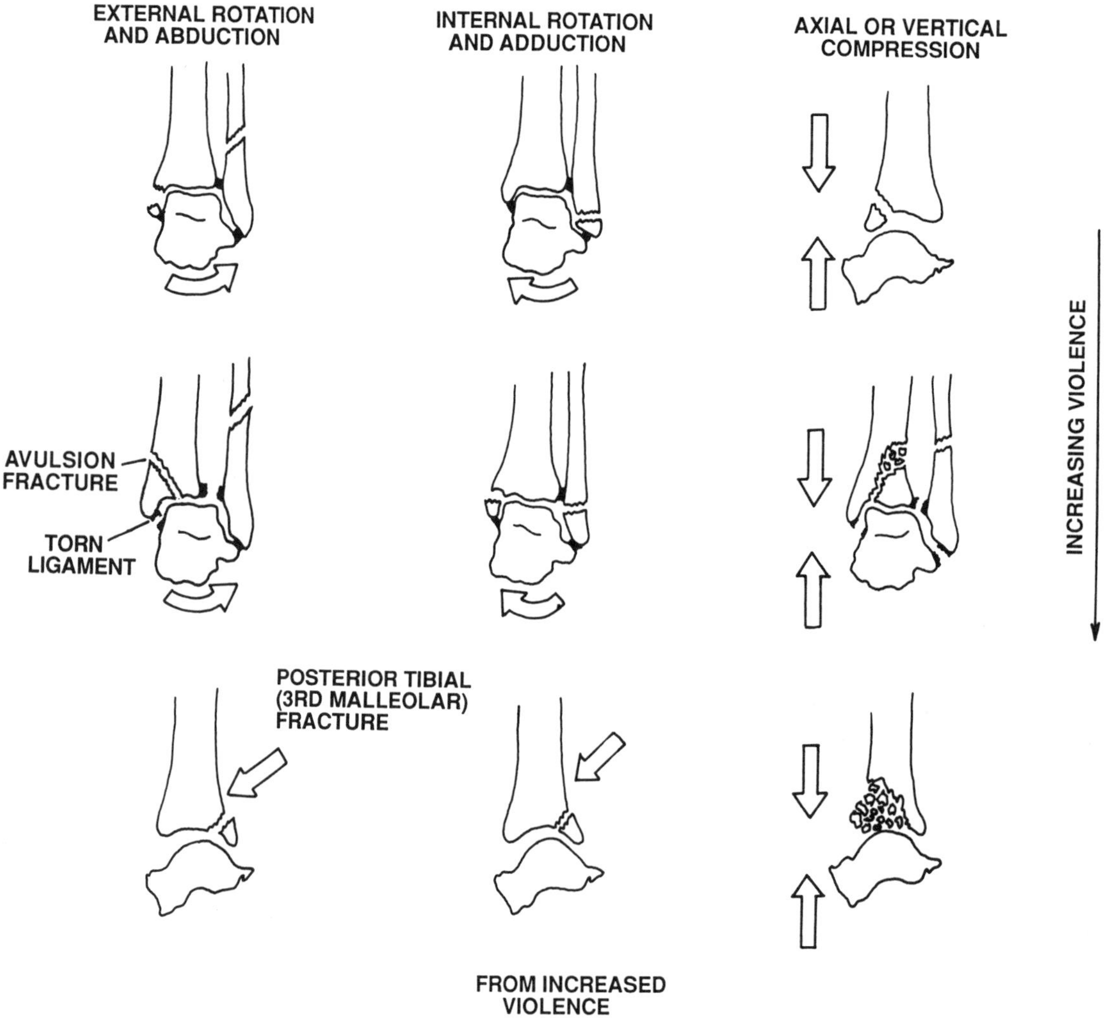

Figure 25
SOME FRACTURE MECHANISMS OF THE ANKLE JOINT FROM CAR CRASHES

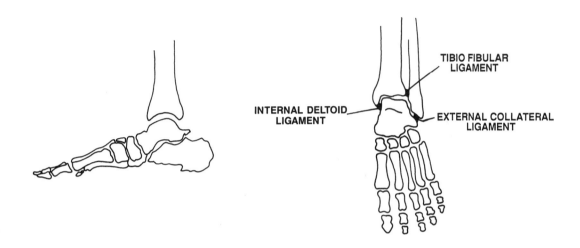

Figure 25
SOME FRACTURE MECHANISMS OF THE ANKLE JOINT FROM CAR CRASHES

This illustration is an idealized presentation of some basic mechanisms of ankle joint fractures. It shows only those bones and ligaments that we wish to show and does not show the many other ligaments of this region that are of less importance in demonstrating fracture pattern causation. The upper surface of the talus demarcates the line of malleolar shear fractures that are caused by the talus. Below the uppermost talar surface most malleolar fractures may be blamed on the mechanism of avulsion ("pulling") where ligaments are attached.

In the less idealized world of vehicular trauma the damage that results from axial compression, as shown at the right side of this illustration, often is combined with the damage that results from rotations and from movements toward or away from the mid-line (i.e., from shear and/or avulsion fractures). In the more violent car crashes we can expect to have the ankle syndesmosis split and the distal tibia and fibula fragmented (comminuted) as well.

As we will see in figure 26 that follows, substantial internal or external rotation at the ankle joint as a result of upward floor pan displacement almost has to have at least some component of axial compression. As can be readily seen above, the combination of avulsion, shear, and compressive forces may cause thoroughly untidy fractures.

and of the clinical import and treatment of the various fractures are references [10] and [11], respectively.)

The stresses that caused specific fracture patterns were shown in figure 14, chapter 3, and they are the key to understanding the long bone fractures that follow, albeit they apply to all other bone fractures as well.

To review in brief: transverse fractures result from bending and tension loadings; spiral fractures result from torsional loads; axial compression causes joint surface compression or impaction fractures. To this we now add *avulsion* fractures, which are fractures involving bone where tendon or ligament is attached and which are due to tendons or ligaments being put into tension and tearing off the bony attachment sites.

Figure 25 shows three major fracture mechanisms and patterns for the ankle joint. It considers three malleoli: the medial (tibial) malleolus, the lateral (fibular) malleolus and then considers the posterior lip of the distal tibia to be a third malleolus.

- **External Rotation + Abduction** - The fractures are often above the syndesmosis.
- **Internal Rotation + Adduction** - The fractures are often below the syndesmosis.
- **Axial (vertical) Compression** - Crushed articular surfaces, often with fragmentation.

Fractures typical for each of the above patterns are given in figure 25, which also shows that as the violence increases, the number of fractures, the number of bone fragments, the number of ligaments torn and the amount of dislocation all tend to increase.

Any and all three malleoli may be sheared off *at or above the joint line* because the talus pushed them off in shear.

Avulsion injuries fracture the involved malleolus *below (or distal to) the joint line*, the fracture fragments having been torn off by ligamentous tension.

Rotation, external or internal, may shear off up to all 3 malleoli, tearing a ligament or two in the process. We would call these "malleolar, bimalleolar and trimalleolar" fractures.

Abduction may shear the lateral malleolus and avulse the medial malleolus.

Extreme axial compression, especially with the foot dorsiflexed, may cause so called "pylon" fractures, (may also be spelled "pilon"), in which the distal end of the tibia will either split or shatter, completely disrupting the ankle.

It is not difficult to see how these directions of force would be applied in collisions, and figure 26 shows how buckling the floor pan or toe pan could cause different fractures according to where the foot happens to be at the moment of buckling.

I would like to have been able to discuss with you some crash literature supporting these clinically well known, clinically well studied patterns and mechanisms of ankle fractures, but there are few non-clinical automotive crash injury papers which attempt to define foot and ankle joint injury mechanisms, and few are of a standard that I can rely upon. For example, a recent SAE paper entitled "Human Ankle Impact Response in Dorsiflexion" involved 18 lower limbs from 9 cadavers. However, 12 of the 18 limbs (67 percent) sustained no injury at all; 3 limbs had ankle fractures and 3 limbs sustained sprains only.(!)

I'm sorry, but to me at least, 3 fractures and 3 sprains do not a study of impact ankle response to dorsiflexion make. But from these 3 fractured ankles and 3 sprained ankles there was published some 4 tables and 11 figures, running 15 journal pages, all for 3 fractures and 3 sprains of the 18 cadaver limbs tested. I have little use for conclusions drawn from such data.

Or how about an SAE paper of 1991, entitled "Ankle Joint Injury Mechanism for Adults in Frontal Automotive Impact"? This curious study utilized computer based weighted NASS files to access NASS "hard copy" (the NASS paper report for each injured occupant). Then, without examining either X-rays, X-ray reports, medical charts or the vehicles themselves, the authors "associated" an ankle injury mechanism with each occupant. In short, they published a statistical summary of surmised injury mechanisms for surmised injuries due to surmised vehicle damage, the latter two surmises being derived from NASS report forms, while the basis for surmising the injury mechanisms was not stated. The authors admitted that the NASS report forms did not even report "specific diagnoses" for the injuries.

I have surmised that I cannot use that sort of information, even if two of the authors are from the NHTSA.

The Leg (tibia and fibula)

Table 7 of this chapter gave the distribution of lower limb injuries from 3 "automotive" and one "clinical" article. Of the tibia/fibula injuries which did occur, they varied from about 15 to 30 percent of the lower limb injuries, the higher figure being from the only study which included lateral and rear collisions, the 3 other studies being constrained to frontal impacts. Thus, between 1 of every 3 to 1 of every

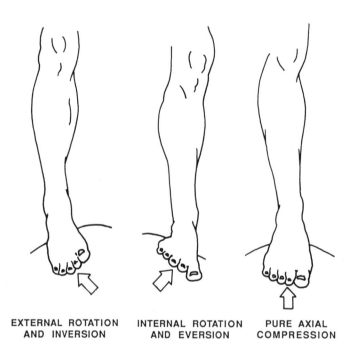

EXTERNAL ROTATION INTERNAL ROTATION PURE AXIAL
AND INVERSION AND EVERSION COMPRESSION

Figure 26
HOW FLOOR PAN DEFORMATION MAY ROTATE AND COMPRESS THE ANKLE

Where the foot is located with reference to the floor pan at the exact time that the floor pan is deformed by a force in plane will determine which direction the foot will be moved. Here we may see how the foot (and the ankle joint therefore) will be moved by the sudden movement of the buckling floor pan.

It may be seen how at least some amount of axial compression will occur as the deforming floor rises under the foot. It may also be realized how the location of the apex of the rising mound of floor pan will rotate the foot depending upon where the apex is located with regard to the long axis of the foot and the ankle joint.

Note that we should expect external rotation to occur in combination with some *inversion* of the foot, that internal rotation will occur with *eversion* of the foot, and that both occur with a variable amount of axial compression.

7 or 8 lower limb injuries is an injury to the tibia and/or fibula. Fortunately, for frontal impacts at least, closed fractures of the tibia/fibula are 5 to 6 times more common than open fractures.

While this is true for automobile impacts, the reverse is true for motorcycle and pedestrian impacts; open tibia/fibula fractures are more the rule than the exception for pedestrians and cyclists. It might also be worth reminding you that motorcyclists and pedestrians are 1 of every 4 or 5 vehicle deaths, which is to say, they are not rare events.

If you reach down and feel either leg just below the knee joint you will feel the tibia, just beneath the skin. And I mean *just* beneath the skin; the bone usually has less than one-quarter of an inch of skin and subcutaneous tissue between it and the outside world. It is not difficult to visualize a spiral or oblique fracture's sharp edges over-riding each other and tearing right through the skin. And not only is the skin covering the tibia quite thin, the membrane containing the blood and nerve supply of the bone, the periosteum, is also unusually thin at the subcutaneous border and therefore lends little mechanical support, tears easily and strips more readily than elsewhere. All of this means that tibial shaft fractures displace more readily, heal more slowly and infect more easily than most fractures.

Most mid-leg crash fractures are from *direct* blows, causing transverse or short oblique fractures, often involving both tibia and fibula shafts at the same level.

Fractures of the middle and lower thirds of the tibial and fibular shafts generally are high energy injuries, and like most high energy fractures, are frequently comminuted.

Displaced fractures of the upper 1/3 of the tibia jeopardize the popliteal artery where it divides into the anterior and posterial tibial arteries, and jeopardize, therefore, the very survival of the leg below the damaged artery.

Finally, the anatomy of the region itself may cause a relatively odd complication, swelling inside of the closed fascial spaces ("compartments") of the mid-leg causing surprisingly high pressure within the compartments which, in turn, compromises circulation to the lower leg and foot. Unless emergently relieved by operative fasciotomy, much of the muscle of these compartments may die and be replaced by fibrous tissue, ultimately resulting in a largely useless lower limb.

All in all, fracture of the tibia, perhaps the most commonly fractured of all of the long bones, is a catastrophe waiting to happen.

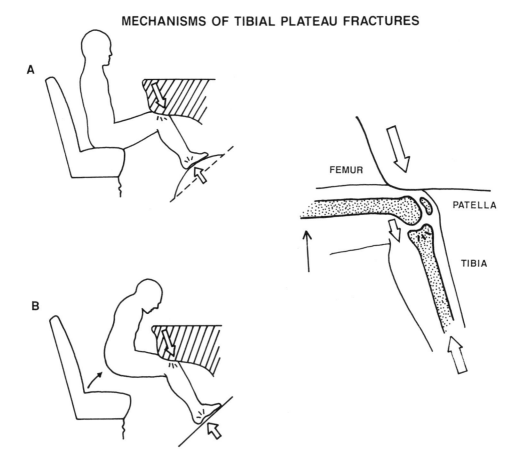

MECHANISMS OF TIBIAL PLATEAU FRACTURES

Figure 27
TIBIAL PLEATEAU FRACTURE MECHANISMS

Shown here are two mechanisms whereby the tibial plateaus may be fractured by frontal car crashes.

Figure 27A shows a front seat occupant who slid forward on impact, entrapping knees beneath the dashboard even as the floor pan elevated (by oil-canning or buckling), thus driving the tibial plateaus up against the femoral condyles.

Figure 27B shows a front seat occupant with knees again entrapped below the dashboard. In this case there is little or no floor pan distortion, but the occupant rises off the seat as he is inertially thrown forward because, although the legs cannot move further forward, the upper torso can and does continue to move forward. The edge of the dash acts as a fulcrum as the proximal femur rises, thus rotating the femoral condyles down into the tibial plateaus.

Neither mechanism would be expected to happen with adequately restrained occupants, although the figure 27A mechanism could still happen to a tall occupant in a small car, whether restrained or not.

Tibial plateau fractures occurring in average or small occupants during frontal impacts suggest that the occupant was unrestrained. I use surrogates in exemplar vehicles to help make this determination.

The Knee

In frontal crashes reviewed in the National Accident Severity Study for the years 1980-87, adult unrestrained drivers sustained 89 percent of their knee injuries from dashboard (instrument panel) contacts and only 4 percent from steering assembly contacts[6].

In an earlier in-depth study of 153 people injured in motor vehicle accidents, there were 80 knee injuries of which 69 were from dashboard contact[12].

The most common knee injury occurs when the knee strikes the dash or steering column in a frontal collision, as was shown in figures 1 and 2 in chapter one. When the front of the knee strikes a small area, such as a projecting cigarette lighter or knob on the dash, or the rigid steering column, the load is concentrated and may cause fracture of the patella (knee cap), a crush fracture, generally comminuted and stellate in shape.

When the knee strikes smooth sheet metal of the dashboard, or smooth plastic with sheet metal behind it, the knee itself generally is not significantly injured, although a fracture of the femur or dislocation of the hip may occur in high energy accidents.

While these mechanisms of injury refer to front seat occupants, they apply equally well to rear seat occupants striking the backs of the front seats rather than striking their knees into the dashboard.

Fractures of the tibial plateau generally are depressed fractures occurring when the knee is trapped under the dashboard (figure 27), and then either axially loaded because of buckling or "oil canning" of the floorboard (figure 27A) or from the unrestrained occupant rising from the seat as he flexes forward (figure 27B). In each case the femoral condyles are driven into the tibial plateaus and condylar fractures may also occur.

About 50 percent of tibial plateau fractures also have associated meniscal cartilage injuries[13].

As with other knee injuries, lateral or medial loads applied to the knee cause medial and lateral collateral ligament damage, respectively. Perpendicularly striking the proximal tibia may tear the posterior cruciate ligament or fracture the proximal tibia.

While intra-articular fractures involving the knee joint necessarily damage articular cartilage, meniscal cartilage damage is another story entirely. For example, in order to tear the medial meniscus, (those tears are at least 6 times more common than the less mobile lateral meniscus[8]), it is necessary to axially load the partially flexed knee while the tibia is externally rotated (with respect to the femur) and then abduct it further, exceeding the normal ranges of external rotation and abduction[8].

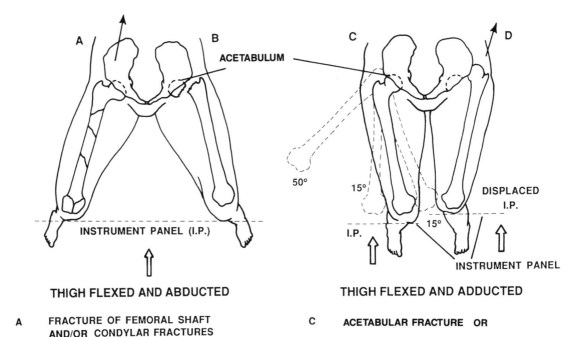

FIGURE 28
INJURIES OF THE FEMUR AND ACETABULUM IN FRONTAL CRASHES

There's a lot of information in these 2 illustrations. A good place to start is at 28C, so that we may note the *neutral* position of the femur (drawn in solid lines) is where the thigh shows neither *abduction* (in the above diagram it is seen drawn at +15 and +50 degrees, or *abducted*, and shown as dotted lines) nor *adduction* (seen drawn at -15 degrees, or *adducted*, again shown in C above as dotted lines).

In the seated position of A and B above, (with the thigh flexed and *abducted*), frontal crash will cause the knee to strike the dashboard, resulting in possible fractures of the femoral condyles, shaft, or head (either intracapsular or extracapsular).

With the thigh flexed and *adducted*, the potential injuries from frontal impacts become acetabular fractures and/or posterior dislocation of the femur, as shown in figure C and D.

When the thigh is flexed and in *neutral* position, either A, B, C, or D may occur with frontal impact. However, pure frontal impact is rare; some degree of rotation from off-center frontal impact is most common, so even the neutral thigh position would be expected to yield either the effects of abduction or adduction, depending upon the direction of rotation that is coupled with the frontal impact.

In short, even the pre-impact positions of the thigh — which should predict the category of fracture in a frontal impact and which are the very distinctions made in the examples above — even they require some thought when applied to any given accident. But then, you probably knew *that*.

Another mechanism by which medial meniscal tears may occur requires very sudden, full extension or hyperextension while under axial load[14]. Unfortunately, there have been no reports or reviews of ligamentous, meniscal or articular cartilage injuries due to vehicle crash[15] so we cannot discuss the incidence of these injuries, although in my experience meniscal tears are uncommon in vehicular crash absent other, more severe damage to the knee joint. States[15] estimates some 10 to 20 percent of ligamentous, meniscal and articular cartilage injuries are motor vehicle related, based on his own (certainly very extensive) experience; the rest are nearly all sports injuries.

While there are no motor vehicle crash studies of specific knee injuries, there are numerous studies of the distribution of motor vehicle crash injuries reported under the lumped headings of the Abbreviated Injury Scale as "AIS 2 or AIS 3." This is a good example of why I have earlier referred to the AIS system as inadvertently having corrupted crash injury literature by its pervasive lack of reporting specificity. To badly paraphrase Omar Khayyam, "I wonder often what using the AIS buys one half so precious as the stuff it sells."

The Femur

The femur is the largest long bone, with a substantial, thick cortical wall for most of its length, but with relatively thin-walled, crushable, cancellous bone at both ends.

The distal end of the femur has two somewhat bulbous condyles that articulate with the tibial plateaus, forming the superior portion of the hinge-like joint just discussed previously, the knee joint. What is unpleasant about the design is that these condyles are thin walled and have a wedge shaped sesamoid bone, the patella (knee cap), that travels in the intercondylar groove as follows:

- from full extension to full flexion the patella glides upon the femoral condyles for some 7 cm;
- from full extension to 90 degree flexion *both* condyles articulate with the patella;
- beyond 90 degree flexion the patella externally rotates, articulating *only* with the medial facet (i.e., the medial condyle).

Thus, when the knee contacts the dash or the steering post in a crash with a significant frontal component, we can expect that the wedge-like patella may be driven between the two condyles, splitting one or both from the shaft (from full extension to 90 degree flexion), and splitting the medial condyle from the shaft when the leg is flexed 90 degrees or more. With the right leg on the accelerator or brake, the knee is generally more extended than flexed, so that the wedge-like patella is positioned in the intracondylar groove, ready to be driven into the groove by dash contact.

The fact is, while knee contact with the dash may do varying amounts of injury to that joint itself, it also may transmit the majority of the impact energy to the femoral shaft, causing the condylar fractures noted above, and/or also causing fractures of the femoral shaft (with considerable comminution when there is considerable force), and fracturing and/or fracture-dislocating the proximal femur as well as fracturing the acetabulum of the hip[16] (see figure 28).

Femoral shaft fractures are about equally common in the upper (proximal), middle, and lower (distal) thirds[11]. The patterns of femoral shaft fractures are quite variable. They are also quite valuable in that we can usually infer the direction and relative magnitude of the causal forces from the fracture pattern; i.e., torsion causing spiral fractures, direct perpendicular blows causing transverse fractures, increasing force causing increasing comminution and so forth, as we have discussed in chapters three and four.

Because the femoral shaft is very strong, great violence is required to produce fractures of the shaft, thus we often see extensive tearing of the periosteum, at least some comminution and, therefore, instability of the fracture. The nearly unrestrained motion of fracture fragments produces relatively massive muscle tissue damage and massive internal hemorrhage.

(I remember a young adult unrestrained front seat passenger brought by ambulance a considerable distance to the county hospital emergency room in Ohio where I was on duty. The victim's only apparent injuries were bilateral femoral fractures — obvious to anyone from the massive distension and foreshortening of her thighs. She was dead on her arrival at the hospital. The record of her pulse and blood pressure changes during transport to the hospital were eloquent proof that the rate of intravascular fluid replacement was insufficient to keep up with the extraordinary rate of blood loss into her own thigh tissues. She had rapidly bled to death into her own thigh tissues. Of course, that was some twenty five years ago, when nearly untrained volunteers manned ambulances in some parts of our country.)

Fractures of the proximal femur, (at the hip), may be divided into two major categories, depending on whether or not the fracture is within or without the hip joint capsule:

- **extracapsular** — either between the greater and lesser trochanters or through them (i.e., intertrochanteric or pertrochanteric fractures). They are injuries of the golden years; they are AARP injuries, most common in the 55 years and older group. Women more often than men endure this injury because of post-menopausal or senile osteoporosis. However, the cancellous bone's generous blood supply assures a high probability of good healing.

• **intracapsular** — these fractures are ominously described by Salter as "fraught with complications . . . among the most troublesome and problematical of all fractures." Again these are most common in elderly women for the same reasons given for extracapsular hip fractures. Perhaps largely because the blood supply to the intracapsular femur is so precarious, only 50 percent of patients so injured have satisfactory results of treatment, which is by far the worst results of any fracture in the entire body[8].

Fracture-dislocations of the hip are uncommon from causes other than crash injury. After all, the hip is such a stable joint, a full ball-in-socket joint, that it pretty much requires the violence of a vehicle crash to force the femoral head out of the acetabular socket.

The pathomechanics of femoral dashboard injuries were well described by 1958[16]. Figure 28 shows how striking the dashboard with the knee when the thigh is flexed and adducted produces posterior dislocation of the femur, with or without fracture of the posterior lip of the acetebular rim.

Necessarily, posterior dislocation of the head of the femur pierces the joint capsule, and therefore, until the dislocation is relocated, the extracapsular location of the femoral head jeopardizes its blood supply. Unless posterior dislocation, with or without fracture, is dealt with emergently, there will be avascular necrosis, which is to say that the head of the femur may die. Posterior dislocation of the head of the femur also threatens the sciatic nerve located at the posterior/inferior margin of the hip joint. The sciatic nerve is the largest peripheral nerve in the body, about two centimeters (over 3/4 of an inch) in diameter, and it really is two separate nerves (the tibial n. and the common peroneal n.) in the same connective tissue sheath. Damage to the sciatic nerve may cause paralysis of the "hamstring" muscles of the posterior thigh and most of the lower leg. Sensory losses from sciatic nerve damage is far more spotty in distribution and of less consequence than motor losses.

Figure 28 also shows that striking the thigh axially when it is flexed and abducted can shear off the head of the femur and/or dislocate the proximal femur. Striking the lateral aspect of the hip, as in a same-side lateral collision, can drive the head of the femur through a comminuted fracture at the center of the acetabulum.

Anterior dislocation of the femoral head is so improbable a consequence of crash, requiring near simultaneous thigh extension while abducting and externally rotating the thigh, that we will here ignore it, going on instead to fractures of the pelvic ring.

Pelvic Ring Fractures

The Society of Automotive Engineers 1986 publication *Human Tolerance to Impact Conditions as Related to Motor Vehicle Design* cites only a single biomechanical study of hip fracture. McElhaney, Roberts and Hilyard's *Handbook of Human Tolerance* 1976 study for the Japan Automobile Research Institute is substantially more complete, but it may be said that "unlike most other areas of orthopedics, there is remarkably little experimental information on the biomechanics of pelvic and acetabular fractures, the bulk of the information comes from clinical observation alone[9]."

The adult pelvis is a large, strong, ring of bone containing and surrounded by important organs, nerves and blood vessels. The pelvis is made up of the sacrum and two "innominate" bones, the latter being formed by the fusion of three other bones in the mid-teens.

This ring of bone we call the pelvis is so strong that great force is necessary to damage it. Great forces are most common in vehicular crashes, so it is not surprising to find that automobile crashes are responsible for about two-thirds of all pelvic fractures[8].

And because great forces are necessary to cause such an injury it is also not surprising to find pelvic fracture associated with other serious, concurrent injuries and, therefore, with relatively high mortality rates, the latter being due to the multiplicity of injuries and to complications rather than to pelvic fracture by itself.

Pelvic fractures account for 1 of every 30 or so skeletal fractures, and perhaps because of associated fractures, have a relatively high mortality rate, variously reported as from 5 to 20 percent[17]. Open pelvic fractures represent about 1 of every 25 pelvic fractures and have a reported 50 percent mortality rate[17]. Nearly 2 of every 3 open pelvic fractures occur in pedestrians; about 1 in 5 are motorcyclists; car occupants represent less than 1 of every 10 open pelvic fractures.

The hip bone (each innominate bone) is formed by the fusion of three bones: the ilium (put your hand on your hip and it rests on the iliac crest), the ischium (it too is not hard to find because that's what we sit upon) and the pubis (which is the firm bulge just above your genitals). The three bones don't complete fusion until near the 16th year, forming a "Y" right through the socket of the hip joint.

ANTERIOR TO POSTERIOR COMPRESSION

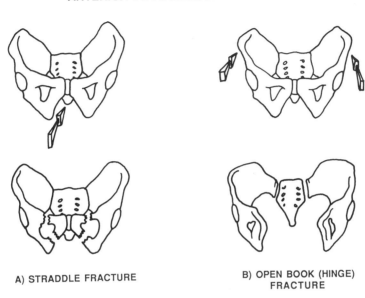

A) STRADDLE FRACTURE

B) OPEN BOOK (HINGE)
FRACTURE

Figure 29
FRONT-TO-BACK COMPRESSION OF THE PELVIC RING

When sufficient rearward directed force is applied to the region of the pubic symphysis (that's the bony region located in front, just above our genitalia) the bones joined there will fracture. We may see some or all 4 of the public rami fractured, as shown in the left side of the above diagram. The same fracture of the pubic rami may also result from a different force, one coming from below the pelvis and directed mostly upward as well as somewhat rearward. Both forces will cause the so-called "straddle" fracture.

When sufficient rearward directed force is applied to the sides of the front of the pelvic ring, as shown in the right side of the above diagram, the pelvic ring may open widely, separating at the pubic symphysis (joint). This "open book" appearance of the separated pelvic ring is termed an "open book fracture," although in some circles it is also called a "hinge" fracture. Note that the open book fracture requires not only that the pubic joint in the front is torn open, but that the sacro-iliac joints holding the sacral plate to the iliac wings of the pelvis are also opened and separated.

These fractures are all unstable, usually have some residual consequences as permanent impairments, and often involve adjacent urogenital structures. They're rather nasty.

LATERAL COMPRESSION

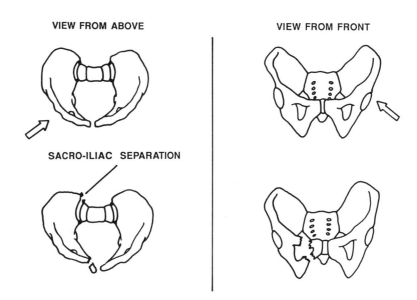

VIEW FROM ABOVE   VIEW FROM FRONT

SACRO-ILIAC SEPARATION

A. IPSILATERAL COMPRESSION FRACTURE   B. BUCKET HANDLE FRACTURE

Figure 30
SIDE-TO-SIDE COMPRESSION OF THE PELVIC RING

When sufficient force is applied to the sides of the pelvic ring and directed in a generally sideward direction (i.e., toward the center or midline) then either of the two types of fractures illustrated above may result.

The fractures that result from lateral compression have an even greater potency for mischief than do the fractures just previously reviewed in figure 29, especially as causes of urogenital damage.

When fracture of the acetabulum occurs (other than rim fractures), the most common fracture will be transverse, and it will be caused by force coming from the lateral aspects of the greater trochanter, dividing the innominate bone (i.e., lateral one-half of the pelvis) at the acetabulum into upper and lower fracture segments. The posterior acetabular lip is the next most common fracture. As described earlier, it occurs as a result of and with the posterior dislocation of the femoral head. The remaining acetabular fractures are relatively uncommon, with names such as "anterior column fracture," "posterior column fracture" and so forth. They even more rarely occur as isolated injuries.

Fractures of the pelvic ring seem to be straightforward events whose pathomechanics appear to be clear:

- **Anterior-to-posterior Compression** — causes either:
    a) a "straddle fracture," wherein the four pubi rami are fractured off the ring, usually from a direct blow to the public symphysis; or
    b) an "open book" or "hinge" fracture, whereby the pelvic ring separates at the area of the symphysis and literally opens up like a book. See figure 29.

- **Lateral Compression** — causes either:
    a) an "ipsilateral compression" fracture, wherein the pubic bone is fractured and the sacrioliac joint is disrupted, both on the same side as the lateral force is applied, or
    b) a "bucket handle" fracture, when the force is applied laterally and inferiorly (i.e., from the side and from below). See figure 30 for these fractures.

All of the above fractures which disrupt the pelvic ring are considered to be *unstable* fractures, and have a fair probability of causing future impairment of weight bearing. The lateral compression fractures have the greatest incidence of bladder and uretheral concurrent injuries.

Of course, I said that all of the above fractures and their mechanisms "seem to be straightforward," and, as is usual in fractures of complex shapes, they are not quite as straightforward as they seem to be. Only rarely do forces align themselves as shown in diagrams, more usually causing injuries with elements of both, say, open book and straddle fractures.

Complications of pelvic fractures are common, often devastating, and include internal hemorrhage (with resultant shock), bladder and urethral tears and injuries to the sacral plexus of nerves.

On the somber note of pelvic fracture complications we will leave lower limb injuries, briefly mentioning hip socket fractures before finishing this chapter with a short note on crash injuries of the upper limbs.

Acetabular Fractures

Figure 28c shows how the flexed thigh, held at different angles of abduction and adduction, will generate quite different fractures of the acetabulum (the hip socket).

Once an injury category with terrible disability implications, acetabular fractures have lost a good portion of their awful reputation because total hip prostheses and replacement surgery have so very much improved their prognoses.

CRASH INJURIES OF THE UPPER EXTREMITIES

This chapter began with a lament about the scarcity of publications dealing with upper limb vehicular injuries. Let me assure you that that is still true here at the end of this chapter, I still have found no published treatises dealing with the mechanics of crash injuries of the upper limbs.

I did find more articles with promising titles, such as "Limbs: Anatomy, Types of Injury and Future Priorities" and "Limbs: Kinematics, Mechanisms of Injury, Tolerance Levels, and Protection Criteria for Car Occupants, Pedestrians, and Two Wheelers," and several others as well. They did have interesting things to say about *lower* limb crash injuries, but there was essentially nothing in any of them about mechanisms of injury to *upper* limbs. (The two titles above were from a School of Impact Mechanics, ICTS, held at Amalfi, Italy, in 1983.)

The International Research Council on Biomechanics of Impact (IRCOBI) which sponsored the above-mentioned School of Impact Mechanics at Amalfi in 1983 has also been co-sponsor, with the American Association for Automotive Medicine (AAAM), of biomechanics seminars ("The Biomechanics of Impact Trauma") held at various resort areas, such as Captiva Island, Florida, and Copper Mountain, Colorado and other pleasant locations. The seminar's notes from these meetings, with their paucity of references for upper limb injury mechanisms, made clear that the seminar authors too had difficulty finding any authority for vehicular impact injuries of the upper extremity.

In the previous chapter (chapter 4) we found, from a variety of studies, that upper limb injuries variously rank from first-to-fifth in frequency of occurrence in vehicular crash studies, the rank varying according to the study's methodology [4] [5] [6] [7]. Thus upper limb crash injuries are of rather impressive prevalence, even if they are largely ignored by most crash investigators.

With this extraordinary limitation on crash injury knowledge as available (rather, not available) from automotive literature in hand, we will briefly discuss the upper limbs, starting with a study from a hospital radiology department, as reported in the Journal of Trauma[7] and previously considered by us in chapter four.

TABLE 8

The Distribution of Upper Limb Injuries in 250 Drivers and 250 Right Front Passengers[7]

Bone	Driver	Passenger
Clavicle	1	39
Humerus	38	76
Elbow	15	1
Radius/ulna	115	44
Wrist	58	2
Hand	22	0

While *this study was limited to unrestrained occupants in frontal collisions in excess of 35 miles per hour*, there is much to learn here. Some generalizations would be that:

right front passengers were at least twice as liable to fracture their upper arm or collar bone as were drivers, and

drivers were twice as liable to fracture their forearm and 20 times more liable to fracture a wrist or hand than were right front passengers.

Because I know of no didactic study to tell us why this was so, (although the above authors extensively speculated as to injury causalities), I shall draw upon my years of emergency room practice to note that it was not rare to find a driver with a bloody mouth and tooth marks (bite puncture wounds, in fact!) of the forearm, wrist or hand. When the mouth was closed and/or the driver's head was rotated, the driver's head would strike the forearm, wrist or hand. With the compliance of the skin of the head and arms being similar one would not except much in the way of bruises or lacerations, but fractures of the bones of the lower arm captured between the hammer of a striking head and the anvil of the steering wheel should surprise no one and may well account for the difference in incidence and location of upper limb fractures between drivers and passengers.

Most fractures of the upper limbs are neither especially complex nor life-threatening, but when they involve joints, blood vessels and/or nerves, they certainly may cause significant disabilities. The remarkable, relatively new "Injury Cost Scale" developed in Germany and reported in 1989[3] lists "closed gleno-humeral (shoulder/upper arm) fracture" and "closed ulna/radius fracture" as the sixth and eighth "most cost-intensive injuries" in terms of "resultant social costs." Yet I could not find a single automotive technical journal article concerned with how these injuries come about in car crashes.

Excepting amputation, the most serious of the upper limb crash injuries within my experience has been that of excessive motion — either elevation or depression of the shoulder girdle — causing compression and/or stretch damage to the rich complex of nerves that emerge at the base of the neck, the brachial plexus. Most common in motorcycle accidents, such injury may result in paralysis of one or both upper limbs.

SUMMARY

We noted early that extremity injuries probably accounted for more injuries and more disability than any of the other body regions.

We also noted that the lower limbs have received some study and the upper limbs about none at all, at least with regard to their mechanisms of injury.

With respect to amelioration of extremity injuries, the limbs are not themselves restrained and, except for only occasional design and installation of knee bolsters, nothing much is done by way of interior padding to reduce injury to these regions of the body most often injured in crash.

BIBLIOGRAPHY

1. Guyon, M.A. and J.C. Honet: Carpal tunnel syndrome or trigger finger associated with neck injury in automobile accidents. *Arch Phys Med Rehabil 58*:325-327, 1977.
2. Levine, R.S.: A review of the long-term effects of selected lower limb injuries. *SAE* paper 860501, and in *Biomechanics and Medical Aspects of Lower Limb Injuries. SAE* P-186, 1986.
3. Zeidler, F., Pletschen, B., Mattern, B., Alt, B., Miksch, T., Eichendorf, W. and S. Reiss: Development of a new injury cost scale. *33rd Annual Proceedings AAAM*, 1989.
4. Pattimore, D., Ward, E., Thomas, P. and M. Bradford: The nature and cause of lower limb injuries in car crashes. *SAE* paper 912901, 1991.
5. Gloyns, P.F., Hayes, H.R.M., Rattenbury, S.J., Thomas, P.D., Mills, H.C. and D.K. Griffiths: Lower limb injuries to car occupants in frontal impacts. *Proc. 4th IRCOBI*, 1979.
6. Huelke, D.F., Compton, T.W. and C.P. Compton: Lower extremity injuries in frontal crashes: injuries, locations, AIS and contacts. *SAE* paper 910811, 1991.
7. Daffner, R.H., Deeb, Z.L., Lupetin, A.R. and W.E. Rothfus: Patterns of high-speed impact injuries in motor vehicle occupants. *J Trauma 28*:4 p. 498-501, 1988.
8. Salter, R.B.: *Textbook of Disorders and Injuries of the Musculoskeletal System.* 2nd Ed. Williams & Wilkins, Baltimore, 1983.
9. Gozna, E.R. and I.J. Harrington: *Biomechanics of Musculoskeletal Injury.* Williams & Wilkins, Baltimore, 1982.
10. Kozin, S.H. and A.C. Berlet: *Handbook of Common Orthopaedic Fractures.* Medical Surveillance Inc., West Chester, 1989.
11. Adams, J.C.: *Outline of Fractures.* 9th Ed., Churchill Livingstone, Edinburgh, 1987.
12. Nagel, D.A., Burton, D.S. and J. Manning: The dashboard knee injury. *Clin Orthop 126*:203-208, 1977.
13. Schulak, D.J. and D.R. Gunn: Fractures of the tibial plateau. *Clin Orthop 109*:166-177, 1975.
14. Sinton, W.A.: Knee injuries, Part 1, the torn meniscus. *J Sports Med 1*:1, p. 37-40, 1972.
15. States, J.D.: Adult occupant injuries of the lower limb. *SAE* paper

861927, and in *Biomechanics and Medical Aspects of Lower Limb Injuries. SAE* P-186, 1986.

16. Ritchey, S.J., Schonholtz, G.J. and M.S. Thompson: The dashboard femoral fracture. *J Bone and Joint Surg [Am] 40-A*:6, p. 1347-1358, 1958.

17. Rothenberger, D., Velasco, R., Strate, R., Fischer, R.P. and J.F. Perry, Jr.: Open pelvic fracture: a lethal injury. *J Trauma 18*:3, p. 184-187, 1978.

18. Judet, R. and J. Judet: Fractures of the acetabulum: classification and surgical approaches to open reduction. *J Bone Joint Surg [Am] 46A*: 1615-1646, 1964.

CHAPTER 6

CRASH INJURIES OF THE ABDOMEN

WHAT EXACTLY IS AN ABDOMEN?

When I here speak of the abdomen I don't really mean the abdomen at all: I actually mean the peritoneal cavity.

When anatomists say "abdomen," they are referring to the cavity bounded above by the muscular diaphragm and below by the brim of the pelvis[1] [2]. But the brim of the pelvis is only a landmark boundary and not a functional boundary — rather like the boundary between the United States and Canada, which is just a line on a map, and not at all a real boundary, as is, say, that between the United States and Cuba, which is ninety miles more or less of very deep water. Now that's a real boundary.

So when I say "abdomen" in this book I mean "peritoneal cavity," and I will tell you why this is so shortly.

Okay. So what is a peritoneal cavity?

Well, I hate to say it, but the peritoneal cavity is best defined as that body cavity bounded (lined) on all sides by parietal peritoneum; this is shown in figure 31, and its bounds are defined:

above - by the diaphragm, a muscular wall between the abdomen and the chest cavities and through which passes major blood vessels, nerves and the esophagus;

below - and anterior by the urogenital diaphragm, a muscular wall across the outlet of the pelvis and through which passes the vagina/penis, and posteriorly by the anal triangle, through which passes the rectum;

in front - by the anterior abdominal muscles (the internal and external oblique and the rectus muscles);

in back - by the pancreas, a segment of the small intestine (the duodenum), kidneys, ureters, suprarenal glands, the quadratus lumborum, iliacus, and psoas muscles, nerve

THE PERITONEAL (TRUE ABDOMINAL) CAVITY

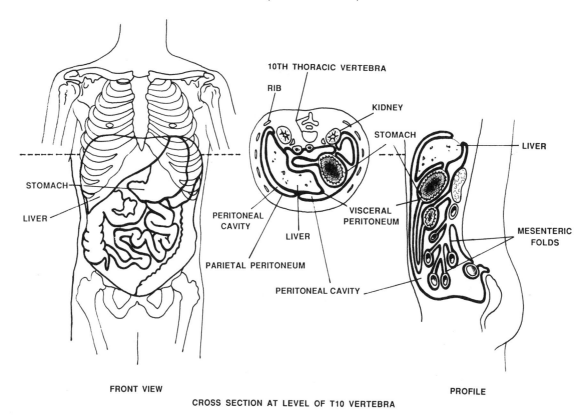

FRONT VIEW

CROSS SECTION AT LEVEL OF T10 VERTEBRA

PROFILE

Figure 31
THE PERITONEAL CAVITY (THE "TRUE" ABDOMINAL CAVITY)

Above are frontal, side, and cross-section views of the abdominal cavity.

The frontal view shows that the abdominal cavity occupies about 3/4 of the entire trunk. To put it otherwise, we see that only the first 4 or 5 ribs are the outer bounds of the chest. The remaining lower 7 ribs largely shield the upper 1/2 of the abdominal (peritoneal) cavity, including most of the liver, spleen and much of the stomach (although a sliver of lung does reach down on the periphery to the lower ribs).

The entire abdominal cavity (as it is defined in the text) is seen here lined with a thin, tough membrane termed the "parietal peritoneum", which is reflected on itself to also cover all apparent contents of the cavity. In addition to all solid and hollow viscus covered by the reflected membrane, this "visceral peritoneum" has other names, such as "mesenteric folds" or "mesentery", where it may perhaps have seemed appropriate to ancient anatomists to create these additional names. Whatever it is termed, it is still just one big, continuous, peritoneal cavity.

trunks and ganglia of the autonomic nervous system, the aorta and vena cava and their pelvic divisions, and the vertebral body column;

on the sides - largely by the transverse and oblique abdominal muscles, but at the upper portion, also by the lower ribs and intercostal muscles.

Hopefully, figure 31 should make all of this a lot more clear than just talking about it.

The visceral contents of this "abdominal/peritoneal" cavity are covered by the same membrane as is the inner lining of the cavity, a white membrane that reminds me of the familiar, white, relatively tough membrane between the shell and contents of an ordinary chicken egg, although the peritoneum is rather thicker.

The whitish tough egg-like membrane is the parietal peritoneum. (The word "paries" is from the Latin word for wall, and in biology refers to the lining of any cavity. The term "peritoneum" is derived from two Greek words, and means to "stretch about," which is not at all a bad descriptor for this membrane.)

When this membrane lining the peritoneal cavity, the "parietal peritoneum," is reflected back on itself to also cover the viscera that are the contents of the cavity, the membrane is called the "visceral peritoneum" (again, see figure 31). Whether it covers the cavity walls or the visceral organs within the cavity, the peritoneal membrane is slick and smooth and secretes a small amount of fluid — the peritoneal fluid — which lubricates the viscera as they slide against and over each other and against and over the parietal peritoneal walls.

WHY WE SAY "ABDOMINAL CAVITY" WHEN WE REALLY MEAN "PERITONEAL CAVITY"

Anatomists have structure as their realm; physiologists have function as theirs. Biodynamicists must attend both structure and function, but when anatomists create artificial divisions of a single continuous cavity, such as the peritoneal cavity being divided into the abdominal and pelvic cavities despite their uninterrupted continuity, we cannot respect these nominal anatomic divisions. The pathophysiology of this body cavity defies division into "abdomen" and "pelvis" since both are continuous. This continuity is particularly important because of Blaise Pascal.

Who is Blaise Pascal you ask? Why, he was a physicist, mathematician and theologian who died some three hundred and thirty years ago, although "Pascal's Principle'' lives on. It is a simple principle, stating that **"pressure in a fluid is everywhere equal."** And this principle is enormously important with regard to impact injuries of the abdomen, because **when impacted, the abdominal/peritineal cavity acts like a hydraulic cavity,** as if it were fluid-filled.

If the abdominal cavity (that's what we will call it from here on, although we understand it to actually be the peritoneal cavity) reacts to impact as if it were filled with fluid, by Pascal's Principle that means that *a blow struck below the umbilicus will be felt above the umbilicus with the same pressure as where the blow was struck.* If punched on the left side of the abdomen, the liver on the right side of the abdomen and the bladder on the lower front of the abdominal cavity will both be subject to essentially the same pressure as exists just inside the region where the blow was struck. And so will all of the intervening intra-abdominal viscera, hollow or solid.

CONTENTS OF THE ABDOMINAL/PERITONEAL CAVITY

The abdominal cavity is the largest cavity of the human body. It contains the largest gland of the body, the liver, (at about 2,000 grams, or 4.5 pounds), through which about 1.5 liters of blood flows each minute[2]. I mention that the liver is a huge organ and that it has a large blood flow to make clear that any injury or laceration of this soft and friable organ has the potential to cause a very large amount of blood to leak into the abdominal cavity.

The liver is a solid organ. So is the spleen, a gland very variably sized at different ages. It is largest in the adult, at about one-half a pound and about 3'' x 5'' x 1.5''. Like the liver, the spleen has a rich blood supply and bleeds extensively when ruptured; and like the liver, the spleen is soft and relatively friable. So too is the half pound or so of pancreas a solid organ, in reality being two largely unrelated organs — one ductless, the other ducted — sharing a single structure.

The stomach and intestines are hollow organs. The abdomen then contains both solid and hollow viscera (organs). (This too would rate a "so what" except again for Blaise Pascal.) Since hollow organs contain air and other gases, the abdomen, as a virtual hydraulic cavity, also has compressible gas pockets within it because of the intestinal tubing it contains.

Let me say that there is more than a little such tubing: the small intestine being about twenty feet in length; the large intestine (colon) is about one fifth of the entire intestinal length, or about 5 feet long[1]. We would expect therefore that there is more than a little air and gas in the large and small bowel. In fact, there are about 200 milliliters of gas in the average bowel[3] at any one time, and a lot more than that in a great bubble that normally resides in the upper end (fundus) of the stomach. All of this means that the abdominal cavity, as a hydraulic cavity (incompressible, by definition) with regard to Pascal's Law, has its pressure waves damped by these pockets of gas which are quite compressible. The abdominal cavity's distensible muscular walls also damp the pressure wave.

Except for the mouth and esophagus, the entire digestive tract is contained within the peritoneal cavity or is partly covered by peritoneal membranes.

Except for external genitalia and the urethra, the entire genitourinary tract is contained within the peritoneal cavity or is partly covered by peritoneal membranes.

The abdominal aorta and its iliac divisions, and the abdominal vena cava and its iliac divisions are on the posterior wall of the abdominal cavity, as are autonomic and splanchnic nerves, ganglia and plexuses and large lymphatic channels.

The anterior portion of vertebral bodies also are covered by parietal peritoneum.

And Blaise Pascal's Principle says, in so many words, that when we increase pressure anywhere in this cavity, all of the above organs, glands and structures are subject to increased pressure.

How often then is the abdomen traumatized by car crash and how often then is such trauma the cause of death? Is the abdominal trauma attributed to seat belt usage in car crash really due to high pressure transients distributed throughout the abdominal cavity as Pascal's Principle proposed? Since the anterior abdominal wall is relatively soft, why isn't simple compression at any one portion of the wall sufficient cause to explain all or nearly all of the abdominal injuries? Are there other mechanisms possible that explain abdominal injuries? And what of other factors, such as age, sex and habitus?

THE INCIDENCE OF BLUNT ABDOMINAL TRAUMA IN VEHICULAR CRASH

Because seat belt webbing itself has the potential to cause abdominal trauma, we will look at the reported incidence of crash injury to the abdomen in both restrained and unrestrained car occupants.

Blunt Abdominal Trauma in Unrestrained Car Occupants

In their 1988 report of patterns of injury to front seat occupants from frontal impacts greater than 35 mph, Daffner, et al found that, of 250 drivers and 250 front seat passengers, 13 drivers and 33 passengers (9.2 percent) sustained abdominal injuries[4]. It was less than clear whether or not these numbers included injury to pelvic contents since they also reported 105 driver and 106 passenger injuries of the pelvis.

In 1972, Hossack[5] gave the injury distribution of 500 drivers and passengers killed in early 1970. This preceded mandatory seat belt usage in Australia (which began in December, 1970). Hossack's series had 18 percent ruptured livers, 10 percent ruptured spleens, 2.4 percent torn bowel or tears of the bowel's suspension (the mesentery), 2 percent ruptured the diaphragm and about 1 percent ruptured their kidneys. All of which seems to be small stuff when compared to the absolute incidence of brain injury (45 percent) or crushed chests (42 percent) as causes of death in this same series.

In 1982 Malliaris, Hitchcock and Hedlund introduced the concept of "harm" as a measure of injuries to crash vehicles, roughly defining harm as the sum of injuries after weighting each victim injury according to the economic outcome of the injury, fatal or not[6]. In 1985, using 3 of NHTSA's national files, (2 for injuries and 1 for fatalities), they published an updated paper on "Harm Causation and Ranking in Car Crashes[7]," effectively lumping all of the factors of type of car, crash direction and severity, occupant seating position, restraint use and the like into the harm concept. Their data suggests that the abdomen is the third most "harmed" body region in car crash, after factoring for type of car, crash severity and so forth.

Blunt Abdominal Trauma in Restrained Occupants

Comparing survivable abdominal injuries before and after seat belt legislation in Victoria, Australia, Ryan and Ragazzon found no change in the proportion of abdominal injuries or in the death rate from abdominal injuries, but did find an increase in the number of patients admitted with gastrointestinal tract injuries and with rupture of the diaphragm[8]. The latter is a singular injury that would result from acute abdominal compression (remember Blaise Pascal?) — whether caused by seat belt webbing, (possibly, according to the authors, because of improper location of the lap belt portion of the restraints) — or whether due to steering assembly crush, or to intrusion of vehicle components into the occupant's flail volume causing blunt abdominal trauma.

Having mandated the use of seat belt restraints, Canada also implemented a "Fully Restrained Occupant Study" (FROS), creating thereby a specific data base enabling the determination of injuries occurring despite and perhaps because of the use of required seat belt restraints. (What an enlightened approach that is! Compare that to the U.S.A.!) A 1982 report by Gallup et al[9] for restrained occupant injuries gave an overall incidence of about 21 percent abdominal injuries for crashes of unlimited directions. Unfortunately, again, the report was in terms only of the Abbreviated Injury Scale (AIS), so the incidence of specific organ injury was not reported. There were however some provocative findings:

• restrained females appeared to have a higher incidence of blunt abdominal injury than did males, for both driver and right front locations, and females did appear to sustain more severe abdominal injuries;

• restrained short people seemed to be more susceptible to blunt abdominal injury than tall people (there were no injuries of the abdomen in anyone taller than 5'10'').

• obese people had a higher abdominal injury incidence. (Although 6.6 percent of the sample were obese, 25 percent of those with abdominal injuries were obese.)

The authors felt that strong correlation existed between 1) rear-loading of the seat back by unrestrained rear occupants, 2) the occupant's age, and 3) the occupant's sex. They also noted that rear seat occupants restrained only by a lap belt sustained both a high incidence of abdominal injury and more serious abdominal injuries.

We will further discuss seat belt induced injuries in the chapter concerned with them.

MECHANISMS OF NON-PENETRATING INTRA-ABDOMINAL INJURIES

In 1985, Albert King, of Wayne State University's Bioengineering Center, in a paper on regional tolerance to impact refused to discuss impact tolerance of the abdomen claiming that abdominal tolerance information was too limited[10]. (He also did not discuss shoulder and upper extremity tolerance either, for the same reason.)

However, in the same year, 1985, A.I. King, of Wayne State University, wrote and published the chapter on the abdomen in the *Review of Biomechanical Impact*

Response and Injury in Automotive Environment[11].

In fact, both opinions appear to be correct; there isn't very much in the way of good or sufficient quantitative studies of abdominal tolerance to impact to write a thorough treatise on that subject, but there are enough studies of real interest for both blunt abdominal injury incidence in crashes and abdominal injury impact mechanisms to write a good review article on these subjects, which A.I. King surely did[11].

Mechanisms of blunt abdominal trauma, at least with respect to liver injury, have been reported in 1987[12] and 1988[13], by Lau, Viano and others from the GM Research Labs. These studies used liver injury in swine as the sole criterion of abdominal injury; in fact there were no other intra-abdominal injuries noted. As they had previously determined for the thorax (using lung contusion as the injured target organ), a "viscous injury criterion" was determined, derived from multiplying the velocity of abdomen (or chest) deformation and the amount of compression of the abdomen (or chest). When we have injury criteria such as this, which is a rate-dependent criterion, we are acknowledging that the property of visco-elasticity governs injury production for the time realm of vehicular crash. (Do you remember chapter 3?)

If an injury criterion has been found for the liver, does this same criterion also govern for the many other abdominal injuries? After all, Lau, Viano and co-workers have called it a "viscous injury criterion."

I think not. For one thing, no other intra-abdominal organs were found or reported to be injured in their studies. I do not understand equating liver injuries with the whole universe of abdominal injuries, since that would infer that a) when the liver is injured any or all other intra-abdominal organs are injured, or b) other intra-abdominal injuries cannot (do not) occur in the absence of liver injuries.

Of course, neither of these propositions (a or b, above) is true. Reference[8] reported unrestrained occupant abdominal injuries wherein kidney and spleen injuries both exceeded the number of liver injuries, and also reported on restrained occupant injury incidences wherein spleen, kidney, gastro-intestinal tract and diaphragmatic injuries all exceeded the incidence of liver injuries. A recent clinical article about the changing trends of blunt abdominal injury in seatbelt wearers[14] reported that 27 of 32 patients with abdominal injury had intestinal injury, compared to 8 injured spleens and 7 injured livers, the latter reported as "minor."

I am not questioning that the viscous criterion relates to liver injury, nor am I questioning whether liver injuries can kill people; I am questioning whether this viscous criterion, based on liver injury as an assay of intra-abdominal injury, has any value at all as a predictor of other intra-abdominal injuries, or for blunt abdominal injury threshold, for which purposes it appears currently to be obliquely touted.

Almost 30 years ago William and Sargent studied mechanisms of intestinal injuries caused by distributed area abdominal impacts, using anesthetized dogs[15], limiting compression in some animals and transfixing the ileum in some animals. Their data strongly support both shear and compression as mechanisms of impact induced intestinal injuries, since 1) intestinal fixation caused significantly more intestinal injuries, and 2) intraperitoneal pressures always exceeded intestinal intra-luminal pressures.

In a study of 44 patients with blunt abdominal injury causing diaphragmatic rupture, Morgan et al[16] found concurrent intra-abdominal injury in 60 percent, including 13 splenic and 10 hepatic injuries. Of special interest, to me at least, is the fact that there were 2 cases of concurrent ruptured bladder (i.e., located way at the opposite end of the abdominal/peritoneal cavity!). A similar series of 60 patients, also reported in 1986[17], found concurrent intra-abdominal injuries in 90 percent of the victims, including bladder rupture in 5 patients.

To the question then of "What is the mechanism of intra-abdominal injury in blunt abdominal impact?" I must answer "There is more than one mechanism:"

Pascal's principle — even though the abdominal cavity is a wide tube, relatively rigid at the back — and is relatively compliant in front, on the sides, and on the top and bottom — blunt impact *will* cause compression and a wave of pressure will be transmitted everywhere within the abdominal cavity. Of course, such transmission will be attenuated and damped as the wave of pressure travels by the compliance of almost all of the walls of the cavity and by gas pockets. Witness concurrent injuries at opposite ends of the cavity, at the diaphragm and at the bladder.

Compression and shear — In addition to the tidy study of blunt abdominal trauma reported by Williams and Sargent[15] and discussed a few paragraphs back, Leung and others[18] reported an extensive survey of 1,017 real-life frontal impact accidents with lap/shoulder harness (3-point) restrained occupants. They then compared the real-life injuries to those found in 281 frontal crash tests that utilized similarly restrained cadavers. They concluded that significant intra-abdominal injuries (AIS 3 or greater) most commonly resulted from "submarining," which may be defined as the occupant sliding forward, under the lap restraint. They concluded that submarining is common in frontal accidents and is the probable cause of most (more than 65 percent) of the "serious" abdominal injuries resulting from frontal crash for 3-point restrained occupants. Intestinal injuries occurred *only* in the presence of submarining, which is to say only when there clearly was compression with shear forces.

There are some who say there is no such thing as submarining — B.M. Gallup and his co-authors[9] are of such belief — but they offer nothing beyond their opinions to support their opinions.

I personally have had enough cases with severe intra-abdominal injuries, each including substantial intestinal and mesenteric crush and shear injuries that also had obvious signs of submarining; certainly enough to convince me that submarining occurs and that it is associated with severe intestinal injuries. Evidence of submarining is *often* seen. On too many cadavers I have seen marked bruising directly over the anterior superior iliac spines (ASIS), with an ascending series of diminishing-sized transverse bruises above the ASIS, clearly the result of the seat belt webbing "chattering" up the lower abdomen, toward the umbilicus. An additional transverse band of bruise may also be seen across the hypogastrium about half of the time, but it is the chatter marks above the ASIS that is the apparent witness to submarining. How else could such bruises be formed?

SUMMARY

We began this chapter with a redefinition of what we will call "the abdomen," based on the continuity of the abdominal cavity, extending from the diaphragm at the base of the chest cavity down to the base of the pelvic outlet, the urogenital diaphragm.

Lined with peritoneum, a tough membrane which also envelops its contents, the abdominal cavity may be considered a hydraulic vessel, approximately responsive to Pascal's Principle. Our intent in renaming this cavity was to emphasize that it is a single, large and continuous cavity, rather than two separate cavities, which we feared may be wrongly inferred from its two anatomic names (i.e., "the abdominal and pelvic cavities").

We then discussed the importance of blunt abdominal injuries, noting that although abdominal injuries occur less often than injuries at some other body regions, they are the third most important cause of what has been termed "harm."

We also noted that there is some evidence that sex, size, age and habitus may all influence abdominal blunt injury thresholds.

While the abdomen's impact tolerance has not been intensively studied and is not yet convincingly and quantitatively determined, there are sufficient studies to permit discussion of injury mechanisms, which we found to include: compression, shear, and pressure wave propagation. In addition, there are significant frequency dependent influences; that is, impact and blast injury sensitivity that relates to the viscoelastic properties of the specific, individual organs, such as the liver, spleen, kidney, etc.

BIBLIOGRAPHY

1. Gray, H.: *Anatomy, Descriptive and Surgical.* T.P. Pick and R. Howden, Eds., Running Press, Philadelphia, 1974.
2. Frick, H., Leonhardt, H. and D. Starck: *Human Anatomy 2.* Thiemme Med. Pub., New York, 1991.
3. Ganong, W.F.: *Review of Medical Physiology.* 15th Ed., Appleton & Lange, Norwalk, Conn., 1991.
4. Daffner, R.H., Deeb, Z.L., Lupetin, A.R. and W.E. Rothfus: Patterns of high-speed impact injuries in motor vehicle occupants. *J Trauma 28*:4, p. 498-501, 1988.
5. Hossack, D.W.: The pattern of injuries received by 500 drivers and passengers killed in road accidents. *Med J Aust 2*: p. 193-195, 1972.
6. Malliaris, A.C., Hitchcock, R. and J. Hedlund: A search for priorities in crash protection. *SAE* paper 820242, 1982.
7. Malliaris, A.C., Hitchcock, R. and M. Hansen: Harm causation and ranking in car crashes. *SAE* paper 850090, 1985.
8. Ryan, P. and R. Ragazzon: Abdominal injuries in survivors of road legislation in Victoria. *Aust NZJ Surg 49*:2 p. 200-202, 1979.
9. Gallup, B.M., St-Laurent, A.M. and J.A. Newman: Abdominal injuries to restrained front seat occupants in frontal collisions. *Proc 26th Conf AAAM*, p. 131-145, 1982.
10. King, A.I.: Regional tolerance to impact acceleration. *SAE* paper 850852, 1985.
11. King, A.I.: Chap. 4, Abdomen, in *Review of Biomechanical Impact Response and Injury in the Automotive Environment.* PB87-182168/AS, U.S. DOT, NHTSA, 1985.
12. Lau, I.V., Horsch, J.D., Viano, D.C. and D.V. Andrzejak: Biomechanics of liver injury by steering wheel loading. *J Trauma 27*:3 p. 225-235, 1987.
13. Lau, I.V. and D.C. Viano: How and when blunt injury occurs — implications to frontal and side impact protection. *SAE* paper 881714, 1988.
14. Denis, R., Allard, M., Atlas, H. and E. Farkouh: Changing trends with abdominal injury in seatbelt wearers. *J Trauma 23*:11 p. 1007-1008, 1983.
15. Williams, R.D. and F.T. Sargent: The mechanism of intestinal injury in trauma. *J Trauma 3*:288, 1963.
16. Morgan, A.S., Flancbaum, L., Esposito, T. and E.F. Cox: Blunt injury to the diaphragm: an analysis of 44 patients. *J Trauma 26*:6 p. 565-568, 1986.

17. Rodriguez-Morales, G., Rodriguez, A. and C.H. Shatney: Acute rupture of the diaphragm in blunt trauma: analysis of 60 patients. *J Trauma 26*:5 p. 438-444, 1986.

18. Leung, Y.C., Tarriere, C., Lestrelin, D., Got, O., Guillon, F., Patel, A. and J. Hureau: Submarining injuries of 3-pt. belted occupants in frontal collisions — description, mechanisms and protection. *SAE* paper 821158, 1982.

CHAPTER 7

CRASH INJURIES OF THE CHEST

GENERAL

Crash injuries of the chest are either fatal within a brief time period or not; there are few long term consequences.

Note that this is the opposite of extremity injuries — wherein threat-to-life generally is low, treatment may take months or even years, and disability costs are high.

Almost everything that resides in the chest — such as the heart and lungs — and nearly everything that transits the chest on the way to somewhere else, such as lymph and nerve trunks, the esophagus, vena cava, and the aorta and its branches — very nearly all of these items and organs may be considered vital, which is to say damaging them will often be fatal.

If we again use the concept of "harm causation" as an index, we will find that the chest is the second most commonly "harmed" region in the vehicular trauma[2], after the head/face. For restrained drivers, the chest appears to be the third most commonly injured region, after the head and extremities.

A particularly puzzling but common chest injury occurs to 1 of every 6 persons that dies in a car crash. They die because of a circumferential tear of the aorta, the body's largest artery, carrying the entire output of the left side of the heart. More than half of the time it tears at exactly the same spot. It is puzzling because it has been reported as a non-contact as well as a contact injury, suggesting that restraint use doesn't seem to matter and that one needn't necessarily break anything else in the chest for this artery to tear and for the victim to exsanguinate via the tear.

You may or may not also want to know that, except for a single study done in England more than ten years ago[1], I have found no other field studies to define the crash conditions (i.e., direction and magnitude of forces) that cause this surprisingly frequent and generally fatal injury. There have, however, been a number of laboratory studies of the possible mechanisms of this injury that will be discussed later in this chapter.

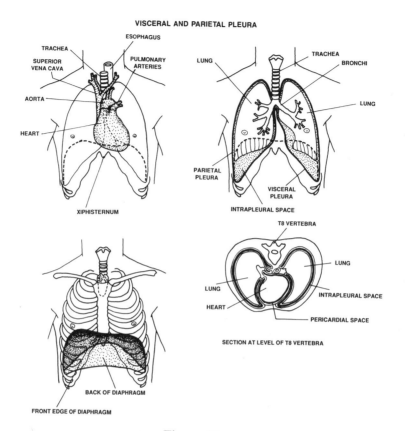

Figure 32
THE THORACIC (CHEST) CAVITY

This illustration is to help gain perspective about the bounds and some of the contents of the chest cavity (also called the *pleural cavity*, the *thoracic cavity*, or the *thorax*). Again note that the bottom of the thorax is just below the nipple line.

As with the preceding figure that showed the abdominal/peritoneal cavity, here we show the chest cavity and its lining membrane, a thin, tough membrane structurally similar to the peritoneum.

As with the peritoneal membrane of the peritoneal cavity, the pleural membrane of the pleural cavity is also divisible into two portions: the parietal pleura that lines the chest cavity and the visceral pleura that envelops all of the organs within the chest cavity.

A distinguishing and important feature of this cavity is shown above in the cross section through the eighth thoracic vertebra, which points out the virtual space that exists between the visceral and parietal pleura and which we term the intrapleural space. This space normally is kept at a pressure below that of the atmospheric pressure outside of the body and its negative pressure is a key element in the normal mechanics of respiration. The usual source for the fluctuating negative pressure within the intrapleural space is the periodic contraction of the muscular diaphragm, which causes downward motion of the diaphragm, increased lung volume and a flow of air into the enlarged lungs. We term this phase of respiration "inspiration" and note here that inspiration (i.e., movement of air into the lungs) will not occur in the absence of negative pressure within the intrapleural space.

THE CHEST (THORAX)

The term "thorax" is the Greek word for "chest."

Most people have no real idea where the chest cavity, the thorax, is located. Most people do have some idea that the chest (the thoracic cavity) is largely bounded by the ribs.

However, as was seen in figure 31 of chapter 6, the upper portion of the abdominal cavity is about at the level of a man's nipple-line, which necessarily also marks the lower margin of nearly all of the chest cavity. In fact, only the upper one-half of the rib cage envelops the chest; the lower 6 ribs largely surround and provide protection for the liver, spleen, pancreas, kidneys and stomach, although there is a near circumferential sliver of lung occupying the gutters of the chest. See figure 32.

The shape of the thorax is that of an approximately truncated pyramidal cavity. It is bounded nearly entirely by the first 6 (upper) ribs, their attached vertebral column behind and the sternum (breast bone) in front. The pyramid's base is the dome shaped sheet of muscles, the diaphragm, which attaches anteriorly at the bottom of the breast plate (the xiphisternum), laterally to a portion of each of the downward pointing lower 6 ribs, and posteriorly, at the levels of the first through the fourth lumbar vertebrae. From about the sixth to the ninth ribs there is a narrow circumferential gutter through which with each breath slides the lowest outermost edges of the lungs.

The chest cavity is lined with a slick membrane quite similar to the membrane lining the abdominal cavity. We give the chest version the name "pleura" (from the Greek, meaning "rib" or "side"). As with the peritoneum in the abdomen, the thoracic pleura not only lines the cavity, it also envelops the organs within the cavity. The portion of the pleura lining the thoracic cavity is termed the "parietal pleura" and the portion enveloping the viscera within the cavity is termed the "visceral pleura." Both pleuras are smooth and glide easily against each other.

In the virtual space between the visceral and parietal pleuras — called the "intrapleural space" — there is a thin film of fluid and a fluctuating pressure that remains below ambient (atmospheric) pressure during all respiratory phases (i.e., while breathing in and out) with the only normal exception being that of a forced expiration. I tell you of this because you should know that any wound of the chest wall which alters this negative pressure prevents respiration, which is to say, stops breathing or makes insufficient the movement of air into and out of the lungs. Such wounds include holes in the chest wall or the fracture of several adjacent ribs (called a "flail chest"). In either case respiration would likely become inadequate and, unless promptly and properly treated, such wounds are lethal.

The thoracic cavity is divided into right and left sides by a rather unsubstantial vertical partition of reflected pleura and loose connective tissue named the "mediastinum" (from the Latin "medius," meaning to be in the middle). The space within the mediastinum is crowded with a variety of organs, nearly all of which are vital, such as the heart and its great vessels, and a few of which are merely interesting, such as the thymus gland.

The esophagus passes down from the neck through the posterior mediastinum and perforates the diaphragm to enter the abdominal cavity. The trachea lies just in front of and against the esophagus before dividing into its bronchial branches relatively high within the chest. There are literally a host of other large blood vessels, lymph ducts and glands, nerves and nerve trunks that also traverse the chest in a north-south (i.e., vertical) direction, within the mediastinum. Again, refer to fig. 32 and/or to any anatomy text or atlas for help in visualizing this region.

While you have out your anatomy book you may want to look more closely at the first 1 or 2 ribs, comparing them to, say, the seventh or eighth ribs. You will find the first 2 ribs to be not only very short as compared to lower ribs, they are also very much thicker than the lower ribs, all of which tells us that it should be a lot more difficult to break the first few ribs — which we found to be very short and thick — than the lower ribs, which are long, narrow, and curved. The presence of fractures of the first 2 ribs thus suggests a more than usual violent chest injury.

The lungs, which occupy the majority of the chest cavity volume, are little more than a network of highly ramified blood vessels running from the right heart (i.e., the right atrium/ventricle complex) to the left heart (the left atrium/ventricle complex), combined with another highly ramified network of air tubes with terminal clusters of micro-air chambers. It is in these microscopic bubble-like chambers that gas exchange occurs between the lungs' capillary blood vessels and the air being brought in and out of the lungs through highly branched tubes.

The blood circulating through the lungs is in a relatively low pressure system as compared to the blood circulating elsewhere, the mean pulmonary blood pressure being about one-sixth that of the mean pressure within the systemic circulatory system.

In fact, there are only 2 to 3 cells' thickness separating the blood inside pulmonary capillary blood vessels from the air within the lung's 3 hundred million or so chambers wherein gas exchange occurs, (termed "alveoli" — Latin, again for the diminutive form of "alveus," or "a small hollow chamber"). The surface area of these tiny chambers provides an enormous surface for gas exchange, some 70 square meters, or about 750 square feet[3]!

This aggregate of millions of blood vessels, millions of alveoli and the airways leading to the aveoli, all that is lung and so necessary for respiratory gas exchange, also and incidentally provides a spongy, packing-like support for the mediastinum and its contents, all of which are captured between the 2 lungs.

Mechanically, having lung tissue against and on each side of the mediastinum is equivalent to packing the chest cavity with soft foam, or tiny bubble packs, in order to give protection to the mediastinal contents during handling or shipping, or even during shaking and knocking about. What a fine economic design! Respiration and impact protection from the same equipment!

THORACIC INJURIES CAUSED BY BLUNT TRAUMA

We will begin here with what could be a way to end this section: ". . . thoracic response is highly rate sensitive. Viscous and inertial forces dominate the initial response, and elastic forces become significant only as large deflections of the system occur."

What Melvin, Hess and Weber[4] have said in the quotation above is that *the rate of application* of force as well as *the amount* of force as well as *the resultant deflection* of the chest wall — all of these factors determine the chest's injury response to force. Visco-elastic properties, as discussed in chapter 3, dominate the chest's response. The probability of injury to the chest or its contents appears to be dependent upon the time period over which a given force is applied to the chest as well as to the absolute amount of force applied. In short, for different rates of application of force, different injury will occur even if the same absolute amount of force was applied each time.

The vital events going on in the chest are both *respiratory*, — the total gaseous exchange between the blood and atmosphere, and *circulatory* — the pressurization of the arterial piping network carrying blood to the various body tissues by the pumping heart. We will therefore separately consider thoracic injuries to the respiratory apparatus and to the circulatory apparatus, necessarily admixing clinical with biomechanical information, even while tacitly recognizing that we cannot damage lung tissue without also damaging the blood vessels within the lung.

Blunt Injuries of the Thoracic Respiratory Apparatus

We will omit discussion of injuries of the respiratory system's upper airways, such as the nose, mouth, larynx, etc. and confine our interest to respiratory elements of the chest. We should, however, remain alert to the fact that some people die because of upper airway obstructions. In fact, Hossack, who personally performed autopsies on some 500 fatal road accident victims[5], noted that *1 out of every 14 deaths was due to asphyxiation following aspiration (the inhaling into the lungs) of blood and/or vomit in victims devoid of any other significant injury.*

The movement of air into the chest requires muscular effort by the diaphragm's contraction and/or by accessory muscles of respiration, the latter also enlarging the chest (and thereby drawing in air) by elevating the downward pointing curved ribs. Clearly, anything injuring the diaphragm's ability to contract, such as damage to the phrenic nerve which innervates that sheet of muscle, or to the muscles or bones of the chest wall, such as multiple adjacent rib fractures, will inhibit or cause the cessation of air movement into and out of the thorax. We call such air movement "breathing," and sufficient marked reduction or absence is, of course, fatal.

Earlier in this chapter we spoke of the virtual space between the visceral and parietal pleura and of the pressure within this space, normally kept below the pressure of the atmosphere outside the chest. When this space fills partly or completely with air, blood or a mixture of these (termed "pneumothorax, hemothorax and pneumo-hemothorax," respectively) the lung on the side of the chest with the leaking air or blood cannot expand fully or at all, depending on the amounts of the leaking air or blood involved.

The presence of air in the intrapleural space is of course related to tears of the airways or chest wall; the presence of blood because of tears of blood vessels; the presence of both air and blood to torn lung tissue involving both airways and blood vessels. Prompt removal of air and/or blood is accomplished by inserting chest tubes into the intrapleural space and maintaining the pressure there negative to atmospheric pressure, an emergency procedure which is often life-saving.

Continuing to move centrally, from the chest wall to the lung itself, the lung tissue which I earlier described as also functioning as a packing material for protection of the mediastinal contents — primarily the heart and great vessels — the lung tissue itself is often bruised (contused, concussed) in a crash, setting in motion a cascade of sequential and often dire events.

The contused lung occurs invariably when multiple ribs are fractured and often even in the absence of rib fractures. (To me the question is "How much?" and not "whether" there is contused lung whenever several ribs are fractured, particularly when the ribs are adjacent.) Radiologic evidence of contused lung is often immediate, and usually precedes the functional loss of lung, the latter becoming obvious by 24 to

48 hours after the injury occurred, when the blood no longer carries as much oxygen.

No, the blood hasn't been altered; the blood carries less oxygen because the oxygen cannot traverse the thickened, swollen walls of damaged alveoli, cannot as easily pass into the blood vessels through the alveolar walls.

Local control of regional blood flow causes blood crossing from the right to the left heart to by-pass damaged lung tissue. This alveolar by-pass is termed "shunting." It causes the dilution of arterial blood with non-oxygenated blood, which in turn reduces the amount of oxygen in arterial blood being brought to other body tissues.

The by-passed lung tissue with its lowered tissue oxygen is itself more vulnerable to infection, with resultant pneumonias a common complication of lung contusion. In addition, alveoli in entire segments of lung may collapse, a condition termed "atelectasis" which causes further shunting and a decreased amount of oxygen in circulating arterial blood.

Brain tissue, particularly injured brain tissue, is exquisitely and adversely sensitive to low oxygen pressures, to decreases in the blood's partial pressure of oxygen. Brief decreases of oxygen going to the brain — even for time periods measured only in minutes — may significantly reduce the brain's ability to recover from mechanical trauma. Thus concurrent lung injuries directly and adversely effect brain injuries.

The preceding sequence of events is not only both dire and dreary, it is frequently terminal, the final pathophysiologic insult to a multiply injured crash victim being that of tissue oxygen deprivation to injured tissues.

Blunt Injuries of the Thoracic Circulatory Apparatus

In the 500 road accident deaths autopsied by Hossack[5] 1 of every 3 victims had torn lung tissue. But 1 of every 4 deaths occurred because of injured major organs of circulation; the heart, the aorta or other major blood vessels in the chest were torn or ruptured.

Dow[6] estimated that 10 percent to 15 percent of fatal vehicular accidents are due to myocardial (heart muscle) rupture and that 10 percent to 30 percent of the victims with these injuries survived long enough to reach a treatment facility of some sort.

Liedtke[7] has emphasized that while non-penetrating cardiac injuries are very common, they are also commonly missed even in the trauma hospital setting, noting that the diagnosis is usually difficult. He quoted Philadelphia's Medical Examiner (in 1966) as having stated that traumatic cardiac damage was the most common unsuspected visceral injury responsible for death and that torn heart muscle was the lesion found most often at autopsy in fatalities due to non-penetrating chest trauma. The ruptured heart muscle was located, in order of frequency, at the: 1) right ventricle, 2) left ventricle, 3) right atrium and 4) left atrium.

Remember too that cardiac trauma includes tears of the septum between the chambers, tears of valves and of the supporting valvular elements (e.g., chordae tendinae and papillary muscles).

The consequences of tears of the connective tissue sheath surrounding the heart — the pericardium — are not known for survivors of the lesion, but Parmley[8] found 13 percent of 546 autopsies did have pericardial disruptions.

A number of clinical investigators have empirically noted and reported that internal damage to the chest is less when external chest damage is greater; e.g., the presence of fractured ribs seems to *reduce* the chance of heart damage. For example, Dunseth and Ferguson[9] reported on 17 cases of ventricular septal rupture in which only 5 victims sustained sternal or rib fractures. I know of no comparable conclusions from the world of crash studies, including that of Newman and Jones[10], wherein, for frontal collisions, both restrained and unrestrained occupants showed an increase in "mediastinum" injuries (defined here as heart, pericardium and major vessels) when rib injuries increased and a decrease in mediastinum injuries when the rib injuries decreased.

As discussed in the beginning of this chapter, 1 of every 6 or 7 crash fatalities is due to aortic rupture[1,11,12]. Well over half of these tears occurs at the same site, about 2.5 centimeters distal to the emergence of the subclavian artery, on the isthmus of the aorta. Even more specifically, the tear is circumferentially aligned, on the anterior and inferior aspect of the vessel. There are many theories and explanations available in the literature[12], but none are so persuasive as to rule over the others.

In my own experience I have seen ruptured aortas in victims that ranged from an 18 year old bull-necked weight-lifting boy who had just received a football scholarship to a 70 or so year old fragile lady. The delta v's neet not be terribly high. In the only field study I've found, Newman and Rastogi[1] reported a mean velocity change of 38 miles per hour, with a two standard deviations' range from about 26 to 51 miles per hour. Collision directions ranged from frontal and side collisions to rollovers, but the frontal collisions were not head-on, and ranged from 30 degrees to the nearside to 60 degrees to the farside. Because none of the impacts were pure frontal, all of the subjects had forces exerted upon them that were oblique to transverse, suggesting a component of shear was required.

As Viano[12] reports in his review of the subject, the aorta has complex characteristics, being 1) non-linear (stiffening with stretch), 2) anisotropic (responds differently when stretched in different directions), 3) is strain rate sensitive (here we go again with that Silly Putty property).

When I put together what is known of the aorta's passive dynamic mechanical characteristics, and what is known of the reported location(s) at which it tears, and what is known of its changing properties as the pressure within it changes, and what is known of the field conditions for the accidents in which it tears (and that usually only one of several occupant aortas tear in an accident in which all were subject to essentially the same inertial forces) — when all of that is considered, the event seems almost like a crap-shoot, a chance event. That is, it would seem that for the aorta to tear, the heart is probably in a specific phase of its cycle (full? emptying? maximum blood pressure?) and the neck held at just such an angle (to put the isthmus at maximum stretch?) and the direction of force just so, with regard to where the aorta changes from an untethered (within the pleural space) to a tethered location (outside of the parietal pleura). Why else should one occupant's aorta tear and the occupant seated beside him not tear, in an event as common as 1 of every 6 car impact deaths?

Cardiopulmonary Injuries in Restrained and Unrestrained Car Occupants: Is There a Difference?

Not if you use the Abbreviated Injury Scale (AIS) and the results of the study by Newman and Jones[10]. "Serious" chest injuries (AIS 3 or greater), were 22.7 percent of all injuries sustained by unrestrained occupants and 23.7 percent of all injuries sustained by restrained occupants.

On the other hand, while the restrained occupants had more "serious" (AIS 3) chest injuries, the unrestrained occupants had more "severe" (AIS 4) chest injuries, for both frontal and same side impacts.

With regard to injuries of the heart, pericardium and great vessels, they were twice as common for unrestrained occupants in frontal collisions and 4 times as common for the unrestrained occupants in side collisions.

Age did not appear to alter the anatomic distribution of injuries in this study, but sex did. Pneumothorax and hemothorax were twice as common in males than in females, but injuries of the heart, pericardium and major blood vessels were 3 times as common in women than in men, and lung injury was twice as common in women than in men. Let us close this chapter with the observation that both sexes broke their ribs and breast bones with equal frequency.

SUMMARY

We discussed the gross anatomy of the chest largely from the view point of packing so many vital and different tissues into so limited a volume, a volume that essentially ends at the lower portion of the breast bone, the remaining rib cage being devoted to enclosing and protecting the liver, stomach, spleen and other contents of the abdominal cavity.

We then discussed thoracic injuries caused by blunt trauma, dividing them into injuries of the breathing apparatus and injuries of the blood pumping and circulating organs.

Lastly, we compared the cardiopulmonary injuries incurred by restrained and unrestrained car occupants, noting that age was not a factor causing different injury patterns but that sex was a substantial factor, causing a tripling of vital chest organ injuries in women as compared to men.

BIBLIOGRAPHY

1. Newman, R.J. and S. Rastogi: Rupture of the thoracic aorta and its relationship to road traffic accident characteristics. *Injury 15*: p. 296-299, 1984.
2. Malliaris, A.C., Hitchcock, R. and M. Hansen: Harm causation and ranking in car crashes. *SAE* paper 850090, 1985.
3. Tortora, G.J., and N.P. Anagnostakos: *Principles of Anatomy and Physiology*. 5th Ed., Harper & Row, New York p. 564, 1987.
4. Melvin, J.W., Hess, R.L. and K. Weber: Chapter 3, "Thorax" in *Review of Biomechanical Impact Response and Injury in the Automotive Environment*. J.W. Melvin and K. Weber, Eds. p. 116, *NHTSA, DOT* report HS 807 042, 1985.
5. Hossack, D.W.: The pattern of injuries received by 500 drivers and passengers killed in road accidents. *Med J Aust 2*:193-195, 1972.
6. Dow, R.W.: Myocardial rupture caused by trauma. *Surgery 91*: 246-247, 1981.
7. Liedtke, A.J. and W.E. DeMuth: Nonpenetrating cardiac injuries: a collective review. *Am Heart J 86*:687-697, 1973.
8. Parmley, F.F., Manion, W.C. and T.W. Mattingly: Non-penetrating traumatic injury of the heart. *Circulation 18*:376, 1958.
9. Dunseth, W. and T.B. Ferguson: Acquired cardiac septal defect due to thoracic trauma. *J Trauma 5*:142-149, 1965.
10. Newman, R.J. and I.W. Jones: A prospective study of 413 consecutive car occupants with chest injuries. *J Trauma 24*:129-135, 1984.
11. Greendyke, R.M.: Traumatic rupture of aorta. *JAMA 195*:7 p. 119-122, 1966.
12. Viano, D.C.: Biomechanics of non-penetrating aortic rupture: a review. *SAE* paper 831608, 1983.

CHAPTER 8

CRASH INJURIES OF THE HEAD, ITS FACE, AND THE BRAIN WITHIN

GENERAL

Head injury is the first or second most common reason for death in vehicular crash[1][2], depending on the study and its conditions. The head is the most frequently injured body region for vehicle occupants restrained by three-point seat belts[3].

But what is it that we mean when we say "head injury?" After all, a scalp laceration is a head injury, but few if any have died from a scalp laceration. In fact, with its plentiful blood supply, it is difficult to keep the scalp from healing no matter how poorly it is repaired. Is simple linear skull fracture by itself a head injury? Sure it is; but it too by itself is only a trivial injury from which neither death nor impairment is an ordinary consequence.

If you read about head injury mechanisms and head injury tolerance you will soon find that some authors mean brain injury and others mean bony fracture tolerance, even though "head injury" was the subject claimed to have been studied. This is unfortunate since the forces required to cause bony damage are quite different from those necessary to cause brain damage, it being both possible and common for there to be skull fractures in the absence of brain injury and brain injury in the absence of skull fractures. Finally, hemorrhage from torn blood vessels extending from the skull to the membranes covering the brain may occur within the bony vault in the absence of immediate injury to either the skull or brain tissue (e.g., epidural and subdural hemorrhages).

One consequence of inappropriately lumping together minor head injuries, such as simple linear fractures, with major head injuries, such as "diffuse axonal injury" (to be discussed later), may be the appalling regulatory concept of "head injury criterion" (the HIC of Federal Motor Vehicle Safety Standard 208, concerned with occupant crash protection). Here tolerance criteria appropriate to and derived from a few cadaveric skull fracture thresholds was seized upon by NHTSA in 1972 and applied to all other categories of head injury as well. And as embarrassing as has been this simplistic misuse of cadaver skull fracture tolerance, more embarrassing has been the long silence of many members of the scientific community who knew better.

It was fifteen years from the institution of this inappropriate head injury criterion as a "safety standard" used by NHTSA until some organized dissent, at a symposium on head injury mechanism[4] sponsored by the Association for the Advancement of Automotive Medicine and Volvo Car Corporation, in September, 1987, concluded that, "A single head injury criterion cannot hope to describe the threshold limits for all types of injury that occur," and that "The HIC alone is quite inappropriate as a predictor of brain injury for restrained car occupants . . .[4]."

However, I believe it a truism that Federal Regulations are a form of what may be called reverse Humpty-Dumptyism; that once put together, Federal Regulations are almost impossible to ever undo.

Now we will attend 4 general categories of head injury, (3 described by Gennarelli[4]), each having its own mechanical basis, to which we have added facial bone fractures and sensory organ injuries since they too are head injuries and are often associated with brain or skull injuries.

TABLE 9

Head Injury Categories

Soft Tissues
  Skin/scalp
  Blood vessels/nerves
  Sensory organs

Skull Fractures
  Linear
  Depressed
  Basilar

Brain
  Focal (contusions and bleeding)
  Diffuse (concussion and diffuse axonal injury)

Facial Bone Fractures

In addition to the command and control functions of the contained brain, the head also contains organs that detect and delineate light, sound, motion, odors, flavors and also define the body's positional orientation in space.

There are 12 pairs of cranial nerves that emerge at the underside of the brain and go rather directly to sensory organs and muscles in the head and neck.

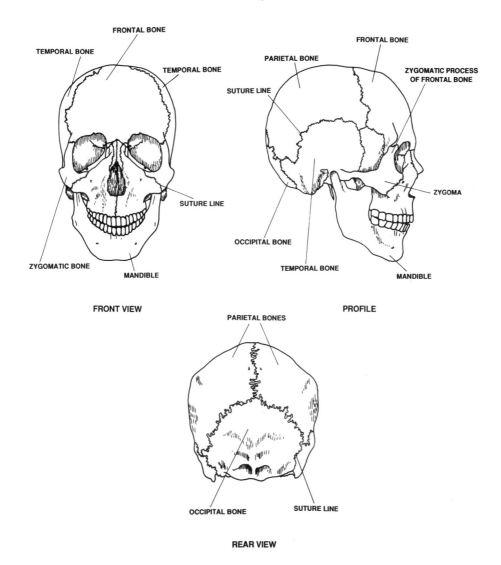

Figure 33
THE CRANIUM AND SOME OF ITS SUTURES

Properly, the cranium has 8 bones. These views show 6 of the 8 bones, the sphenoid bone at the anterior of the base of the cranium and the ethmoid bone located the very most anterior part of the base of the cranium are not visible in this illustration.

In order to show the more familiar appearance of a skull we have included bones which belong to the face rather than the cranium, such as the nasal bone, the zygoma, the mandible and the maxilla.

What I did want to show are the "sutures," the connections (joints) between the bones of the face and between the bones of the skull. As you see above, the sutures are highly convoluted, interdigitating lines of contact between the flat bones and irregular bones of the skull. Fibrous tissue (ligament) connects each bone to the other.

We can consider the head as the:

- entryway for food and drink;
- entryway and exit for respired gases;
- primary location for our sensory organs of sight, sound, balance, motion, taste and smell;
- primary location of communication equipment, from facial expression through speech and sound;
- greatly enlarged anterior (superior) portion of our central nervous system (the brain) which functions to originate or process all motion and sensation, all memory and all thought.

As to such questions that arise when dealing with the central nervous system as "what is the function of the pineal gland?" and "where is the seat of the soul?" we shall leave them for other primers to answer.

So that we may better deal with so complex an entity as the head, we will divide it into 1) the skull and face, 2) the organs of smell, taste, sight, sound and balance 3) the cranial nerves and 4) the brain. Now let us look at each in turn, considering too their injuries.

THE SKULL AND FACE

The skull is divisible into the cranium, which includes the top, sides, back and bottom of the skull, and the face, which forms a portion of the front of the skull.

Of the face, only the bony back of the nose (the cribiform plate), the back of the frontal sinuses and the back of the sphenoid sinus, are in contact with the (anterior/inferior) brain; say less than 5 percent of the brain's surface is in contact with any portion of the face.

The skull contains 22 bones, 8 of which are cranial bones and 14 of which are facial bones. The 8 cranial bones are joined together by immovable highly convoluted joints of minimal connective tissue, called sutures. There are 4 big sutures and several small ones. The sutures all have obtuse names (like "lambdoidal suture" and "sphenosquamosal suture") that you need not know here. Sutures are shown in figure 33, of frontal, side and rear views of the cranium and the face, as well as sutures of the cranial and facial bones.

SIX PILLARS OF SKULL

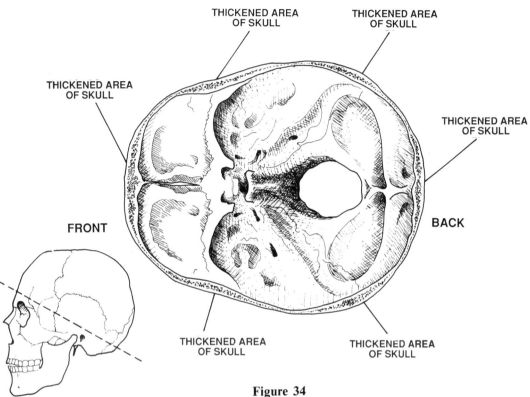

Figure 34
THE PROPAGATION OF CRANIAL FRACTURES AND THE SIX COLUMNS OF THE CRANIUM

In the above illustration there is a sketch of a skull with a dotted line drawn through it, drawn a little above the orbits and above the external auditory canals within the temporal bones. The larger drawing of the base of the skull represents the base as seen after cutting through the skull at the level of the dotted line and removing the upper half of the skull.

When cut this way the skull displays 6 thickened areas and 6 rather thin regions. If we would continue to cut cross sections above and parallel to the present section we would find that the 6 thicker sections and the 6 thinner sections would tend to disappear as variations in skull thickness as we move upwards, toward the top of the skull (the vertex of the skull).

These thickenings are associated with the superior sagittal sinus anteriorly and posteriorly and with extensions of the greater wing of the sphenoid bone anterolaterally and of the petrous portion of the temporal bone posterolaterally.

While it is true that fracture lines may on occasion cross the thickened regions, (and that is most often true of basilar skull fractures), it is also *generally* true that fractures will tend to stay within the thinner sections of the skull, to stay within the paths of least resistance. Let me again emphasize that these variations in the thickness of the skull exist primarily in the base of the skull and in a band extending about four inches above the dotted line shown in this and in the following illustration.

FRACTURES OF THE SKULL

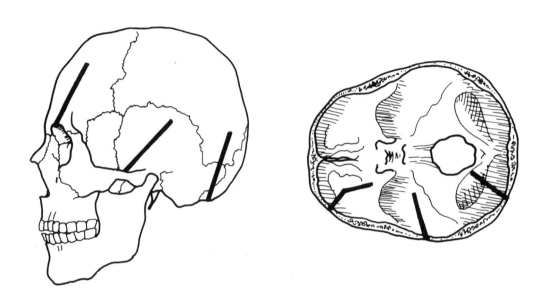

Figure 35
THE "PREFERRED LOCATIONS" OF CRANIAL FRACTURES

In his book about *The Pathology of Trauma* (Lea & Feabiger, Philadelphia, 1954) A.R. Moritz showed what he termed "classical fractures" of the skull. The above illustration shows what I term as "preferred locations" for simple linear fractures and for their extensions into the base of the skull. These locations for frontal, temporal and occipital fractures result from frontal, temporal and occipital impacts respectively. They are classical in the sense that they are frequent, and they are preferred locations in the sense that they preferentially occur where the skull is relatively thinnest.

The fractures are diagrammatically represented here by thick, straight lines.

Note that a region exists approximately equivalent to where we would wear a knitted watch cap or ski cap, on the upper and slightly posterior skull, that is largely devoid of thick and thin sections (except near the midline, where the skull is slightly thicker because of the superior sagittal sinus). Linear fractures occur and propagate simply, in all directions, in this upper skull region, near the vertex.

With regard to injury causation, there are some attributes of the skull that are particularly noteworthy.

1) The cranial vault, or the upper portion of the skull which envelops the brain, has a smooth internal surface fitted to that organ. The bones of the top, sides and back of the cranium vary from about 1/6th to 1/4 of an inch in thickness and they are composed of 2 plates of dense compact bone separated by less dense cancellous (red marrow) bone. Cancellous bone, you may recall, is also found at such locations as the ends of long bones, the heel, vertebral bodies and the pelvis, cancellous bone having the important capacity to absorb and dissipate impact energy.

2) The inside of the base of the skull, upon which rests the base of the brain, is not smooth. It is in fact highly irregular. This irregularity is responsible for *the most common site of focal contusion of the brain*, at the orbitofrontal and anterior temporal lobes, (i.e., the bottom-front of the brain) where the brain contacts these sharp edges of bone[5] [6] [7]. Focal contusions of these regions are known to cause subsequent impairment as behavioral and cognitive deficits[7] as well as impairment of memory.

3) The irregular base of the skull also has some 27 apertures, termed "foramina," through which pass nerves and blood vessels. Thus relative motion between the brain and the base of the skull may cause not only the brain contusions noted above, but tears of blood vessels and cranial nerves as well.

4) If we cut the skull horizontally just above the orbits and the ear canals, the base of the cranium would show 6 somewhat thickened regions of the wall of the skull, as shown in figure 34. Fractures of the lower skull and the base tend to stay within the thinner sections of the skull, following paths of least resistance[8], through the thinnest bony plates. Please note that they do not invariably do so and that this is not true for the middle and upper skull, where the differences in skull thickness are minimal. If we think of the skull has having 6 tapering columns originating in the base that then phase out about half-way to the top of the skull, the propagation of linear fractures of the skull may become clearer and, to some extent perhaps, predictable. See figure 35.

Ring fractures of the base of the skull, which are fractures concentric to the largest opening in the base of the skull (the foramen magnum), do not especially respect the thickened parts of the base of the skull in their fracture propogation, but most other fractures of the base of the skull — "basilar" skull fractures — do tend to run parallel to rather than across the thicker portions of the base of the skull[8][9], (the lesser wing of the sphenoid bone and the petrous portion of the temporal bone).

Since we are discussing skull fractures anyway, I'll place a heading subtitle to dignify the discussion and then elaborate a bit on the subject.

Skull Fractures

As we noted above, the initial impact tolerance curve for the skull was derived from 8 points, representing the durations and magnitudes of accelerations that were found to cause linear fractures in 8 embalmed cadaver heads. In the range of 1 to 6 milliseconds it was found not too surprisingly, that brief impulses required high accelerations and longer duration impulses required less acceleration[10]. What was surprising was the subsequent essential validation of that statistically and biologically improbable curve by both additional and more sophisticated measurements and by scaling small animal studies[11]!

A year before I was born, a New York City Assistant Medical Examiner (and Instructor in Surgery at the Columbia's College of Physicians and Surgeons) reported on skull fractures as found in some 512 necropsies[12]. Dr. Vance found that more than 90 percent of the fractures studied involved fractures of *both* the vault and the base, a fact that has surprised me some 65 years later. Less than 8 percent of the skull fractures that came to autopsy were fractures of the vault alone.

Gurdjian and his co-workers seemed confident in predicting the propogation of skull fractures from studying bare skulls coated with a material that defines stress lines[13] ("stress coat," a varnish-like material).

However, recent clinical and forensic studies do not always support such certainty[9][14][15]; rather, they emphasize the variation of predictability of head impact site from studies of actual accidents and victims.

As to the issue then of whether the causality of skull fractures is determinable from the resultant fracture, I go with reference[13], concluding that *most* skull fractures are predictable in a statistical sense: i.e., that a given skull fracture *most usually* has a given cause. Another way to put it is that identical fractures in a group of skulls generally but not invariably share similar points of impact as well as similar directions and magnitudes of force of impact.

How much force does it take to fracture a skull? Well, you know what I'll answer to that — "it depends on what the impactor is and where the skull is impacted" —

but most studies would put it in the range of 750 to 2,500 pounds[16], with simple flat surface impacts in the mid-range of say, 1,500 pounds of force.

The facial bones are considerably more delicate than the cranial bones, and therein hangs another tale.

Facial Bone Fractures

How much force does it take to fracture facial bones? With the same qualifications as above, the range would be from about 150 to 750 pounds, and this includes breaking the jaw (mandible)[16].

Facial bone injuries, generally termed "maxillofacial injuries," include injuries of the *lower one third* of the face (the jawbone, or mandible), the *middle third* of the face, (cheekbone or zygomatic complex, eyesocket or orbit, nose, or nasal and naso-orbital complex, the upper jaw or maxilla), and the *upper one third* of the face, the frontal bone, its sinuses and the ethmoid complex.

While broken facial bones would not seem to have an injury cost (compensation and social cost) comparable to say, a broken pelvis with residual functional impairment, that is exactly what they do compare to, according to a recent injury cost scale[17]. Maxillofacial injuries frequently are nasty, painful, debilitating injuries, often requiring multiple surgical procedures and often resulting in residual impairments, both cosmetic and functional.

Mandibular fractures, like all fractures, are a function of their particular bony form. Because the mandible is symmetrical we can expect that force exerted on one side of the jaw is transmitted to the other side as well. The weakest part of the mandible is at the condyles, just below the temporo-mandibular joints, so we can expect a high incidence of fractures at that location, quite often on both sides because of the symmetry just discussed.

The temporo-mandibular joint (the jaw joint) is another joint that inserts a cartilaginous meniscus between its bearing surfaces, indicating that it, as with the knee and the sternoclavicular joint, is ordinarily and often highly loaded. That is, the compressive loads of activities such as chewing, which are asymmetric loads when we chew on one side and not the other, result in high loading in terms of pounds per square inch and would cause rapid wear and degeneration were the menisci not present to distribute and lessen the point-loading.

(There has been a remarkable and relatively sudden increase in cases claiming acute traffic accident induced traumatic temporo-mandibular joint (TMJ) disorders. I believe

MAXILLOFACIAL FRACTURES

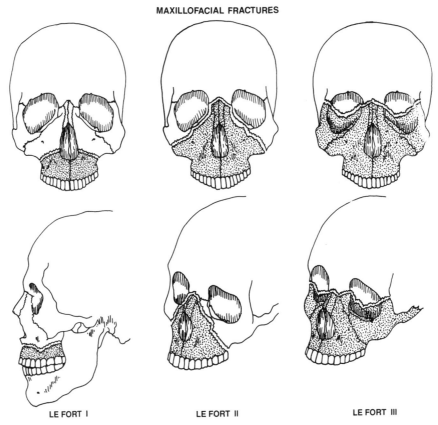

LE FORT I   LE FORT II   LE FORT III

Figure 36
LE FORT FRACTURES OF THE FACE

Fractures of the facial bones may be classified as fractures of the lower face (primarily the mandible, or jaw bone), the upper face (primarily frontal and ethmoid fractures) and the middle face, which is everything else that may be damaged along with the maxilla when the maxilla is fractured. Although isolated facial bone fractures such as nasal bone or zygomatic bone fractures certainly do occur in some car crashes, the majority of complex and severe mid-face fractures that happen are the result of vehicle crashes.

Above are shown the mid-face fractures studied and classified by Rene Le Fort nearly a hundred years ago. The lowered stippled sections show the portion of the maxilla and of associated bones that are fractured along with the maxilla. The enlarging regions of stippling seen above as we go from the Le Fort I to the Le Fort III fracture represents both increasing damage to the facial bones and the increasing amounts of force necessary to cause the damage.

Note that the Le Fort I breaks the palate free from the rest of the skull; the Le Fort II breaks free the nose and upper palate and the Le Fort III separates the entire mid-face from the rest of the skull, also fracturing orbital bones as well as the zygoma along with the zygomatic arch. One need not know details of treatment to realize that cosmetic and functional impairments increase markedly going from Le Fort I to Le Fort III fractures.

that this popular entity should be saved for a book about crash injury mythology, to be combined with rear impact traffic accident induced lumbar disc trauma, the carpal tunnel syndrome and other crash injury tales.)

Maxillary fractures were studied at the beginning of this century by Rene Le Fort and his contribution has been memorialized by the classification of mid-face fractures as Le Fort I, II and III fractures, as shown in figure 36.

Note that the craniofacial dissociation that we term the Le Fort III fractures requires rather considerable force. The prudent and experienced emergency room physician will recognize the typical flattening and lengthening of the face associated with this injury, the so-called "dishpan face," and may look for other, concurrent, high force injuries.

THE ORGANS OF SMELL, TASTE, SIGHT, SOUND AND BALANCE

Were I a teleologist I would argue that the reason we locate sensory organs as close as possible to the brain, the organ that processes the information that the sensory organs bring from the outside world, is that there will be the least time lost in transmitting the data. We may therefore respond more rapidly to the data, should quick response be necessary for, say, our very survival. (You may want to know that nerve conduction is relatively very slow, about a million times slower than the velocity of telephone wire transmission, so the length of a nerve may be significant in its effect on nerve transmission time.) And, were I a teleologist, I would expect that our sensory organs might well be located elsewhere if nerve transmission time were not a factor.

Smell and Taste

Because smell and taste are associated with each other and with eating, we will consider them as functionally together, but anatomically apart.

Flavors as we perceive them are a combination of their taste and smell. When smell is diminished (as in a cold) or lost, as in an injury to the first cranial nerve (CN1, the olfactory nerve), foods somehow taste different, and we may complain that we "can't taste anything," or that "it all tastes like cardboard."

Smells are detected by some 10-20 million sensors concentrated in a patch of mucous membrane of about 2 square inches, in the roof of the nasal cavity, near the dividing septum. Nerve fibers then pierce a thin plate of bone that separates the upper nasal cavity from the base of the brain, the cribiform plate. (The Latin "cribrum" means a sieve, which is what this portion of the ethmoid bone looks like.)

The fibers of smell then course through areas of the brain that facilitate and inhibit nerve transmission to reach the cerebral cortex, the hypothalmus, the limbic system and the reticular formation, which, all together, are concerned (literally) with everything from changes in blood pressure and respiration to instinctual behavior, emotions (including sexual arousal, which may explain some perfumes), as well as fear and rage, the regulation of hormones, salivation and the secretion of digestive enzymes, and, as they say, "a whole lot more!"

This area of the nasal cavity that contains smell sensors also has bare endings of pain fibers from the fifth cranial nerve (CN5) which are stimulated by "irritant" odors and therefore are believed to be responsible for starting sneezing, crying (or at least tearing), inhibition of breathing and other reflex responses attributable to irritant odors. Fractures of the nose and face involving the cribiform plate and associated areas of the ethmoid bone can surely change a lot of things, including and in addition to smell and taste.

Taste receptors are concentrated in taste buds, sensors located on the tongue and palate which, when stimulated, are transmitted via nerve endings of CN7, CN9 and CN10. Again, if I were a teleologist, I might argue that taste discrimination is too vital to risk in a single cranial nerve, since everything tasted is somehow evaluated for say, spoilage or other evils, prior to swallowing. We just can't afford not to be able to have some taste function. Taste has a lot of representation on the post-central gyrus of the cerebral cortex, where its tracts terminate.

Sight

There are four cranial nerves involved in seeing: CN2, CN3, CN4, and CN6. Only the ophthalmic nerve CN2 enters the globe, through the optic canal (along with the artery and veins to the globe); all other cranial nerves enter the orbit through the superior or inferior orbital fissures, which are next to (infero-medial to) the optic canal and 3 or 4 times larger than the optic canal. All of which means that damage to vision may happen because of damage to the cranial nerves serving the eye, either within the base of the skull or as they enter the orbit, with its paper-thin walls and floor.

Eye damage also results from either 1) direct impact to the globe or orbit, often causing orbital "blowout" of the floor or medial wall of the orbit, 2) damage to the orbit from Le Fort II and III injuries and 3) orbital and periorbital injuries from fractures of the zygomatic complex. Finally, damage to the globe from direct trauma is the least subtle of injuries effecting vision.

Injuries to CN3, CN4, CN6 may create double vision (diplopia) because the eyes cannot move in coordination, or cause inability to constrict the pupil or focus the lens (CN3).

Hearing and Balance

Hearing and balance may be dealt with together since they are both served by the same cranial nerve, CN8, (the vestibulocochlear nerve), and they both dwell within the petrous portion of the temporal bone, in a tiny cave-like bony labyrinth that is a replica of the membranous labyrinth it contains. It will be worth your time to consult a good anatomy atlas to see and comprehend just what these odd and delicate sensors are like, should you ever need to understand loss of hearing or balance.

Termed the "inner ear," the vestibulocochlear apparatus has 3 parts, all hollow channels within bone:

- **the vestibule** — a common area of communication between the following two structures,
- **the semicircular canals** — 3 nearly circular tubes at approximately right angles to each other and about one-half inch in size. With two dilatations, the saccule and utricle, this organ provides the sensory input for head position and for the angular (rotational) accelerations of the head;
- **the cochlear** — an odd looking, diminutive organ, about 1/4" by 1/2" in size, it is rolled up like a snail shell, and is the end organ for sound reception.

When basal skull fractures propogate through the petrous portions of the temporal bones there is a real risk of damage to either of the bony labyrinths for balance and for hearing as well as to the canal containing the motor root of the facial nerve (CN7) and the vestibulocochlear nerve (CN8). Should the entire nerve be sectioned then due to fracture involving the canal within the inner ear, then deafness, partial facial paralysis and difficulties in maintaining balance would all be expected.

In the past twenty years or so otolaryngologists have described a clinical entity apparently caused by an abnormal connection, a leak (i.e., a "fistula") between the two very different fluids that bathe different portions of the vestibulocochlear apparatus, the perilymph and the endolymph[18]. It is termed the "perilymph fistula syndrome." I mention this because while it seems obscure, it is being and will continue to be diagnosed with increasing frequency as the triad of symptoms that characterize it become better known.

The triad consists of sudden, often fluctuating hearing loss, vertigo and tinnitus, following anything from blast (such as from gun shots) to mild head trauma and the cervical syndrome (i.e., what some attorneys lovingly term "whiplash").

I have recently seen two surgically proven cases, one from a relatively modest head impact without loss of consciousness and the other with a mild concussion and an occipito-basilar skull fracture. In both of these instances a tiny hole in a tiny membrane in a part of the skull difficult to access has caused serious auditory and balance impairments, permanently altering the lives of the injured parties. The size and location of this injury will make for some difficult cases to try.

The Cranial Nerves

There are twelve pairs of cranial nerves. Some are purely sensory nerves, which is to say that they exclusively transmit information gleaned from sensors back to some portion of the brain. Some are purely motor nerves, carrying directions of "what to do" from the brain to muscle, or other tissues, such as glandular tissue. Some cranial nerves are mixed nerves, carrying signals in both directions, to and from the brain.

It is because damage to cranial nerves is so often concomitant with other head injury[19] that I will here list the cranial nerves and briefly present their functions and, for some of the cranial nerves, their peculiarities.

- **CN1** — the *olfactory* nerve is purely a sensory nerve, carrying "smell information" from the sensors to the brain.

- **CN2** — the *optic* nerve is purely a sensory nerve, carrying information from the retina of the eye to the brain. Some of its fibers cross from one side to the other and some fibers don't do so, so that the loss of portions of the visual fields may indicate the location of the injuries to visual nerve tracts.

- **CN3, CN4 and CN6** — the *oculomotor*, the *trochlear* and the *abducens* nerves are motor nerves to the eye. CN3 serves four of the muscles that move the eye as well as innervating the pupil, focusing the lens and elevating the upper eyelid. CN4 carries motor fibers only to one of the six eye muscles, the superior oblique muscle. CN6 is similar to CN4, innervating a single eye muscle, the lateral rectus muscle.

- **CN5** — the *trigeminal* nerve, has, as its name infers, 3 main branches. It carries sensory fibers from most of the face and oro-nasal cavity and motor fibers to the muscles used in chewing.

- **CN7** — the *facial* nerve innervates the muscles of facial expression, tear glands, salivary glands, taste buds of the front 2/3rds of the tongue and is both motor and sensory to the middle ear and sensory to the skin behind the ear's auricle.

- **CN8** — the *vestibulocochlear* nerve, is sensory to the cochlea to enable hearing and to the vestibular apparatus to enable balance and motion detection.

- **CN9** — the *glossopharyngeal* nerve, is both motor and sensory, and is involved in salivation (e.g., parotid gland secretion), swallowing, taste in the back 1/3rd of the tongue, monitors blood pressure and provides sensation near the external ear. Truly a busy and versatile nerve.

- **CN10** —the *vagus* nerve. As its name implies, it is a vagabond, wandering far, from the palate to the intestines and liver, innervating muscles of the larynx, pharynx, esophagus, smooth muscle within the lungs and slowing heart rate. It carries sensory information from these organs as well as from such select sites as the epiglottis, skin of the opening to the external ear canal and from the covering of the brain in the posterior fossa of the skull. Thoroughly a vagabond, the vagus nerve appears to do everything that all other cranial nerves may have missed doing.

- **CN11** —the *accessory* nerve provides motor fibers to aid in shrugging the shoulders and turning the head.

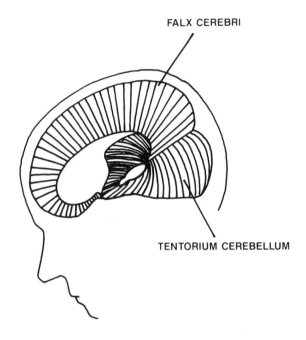

FALX CEREBRI

TENTORIUM CEREBELLUM

Figure 37
THE FALX CEREBRI AND THE TENTORIUM CEREBELLI

During the brain's development the dura folds upon itself, forming four folds that project inward, toward the center of the brain. Some of the margins of these folds contain very large veins, which are also somewhat confusingly called "sinuses". (These sinuses are very different from the collections of air cells or hollow chambers within say, the frontal or maxillary bones, which we also term "sinuses.") The sinuses within the folds of the dura collect venous blood from the scalp, skull and brain, and empty into the internal jugular vein.

These dural folds have biomechanical importance because they separate the cranial cavity into compartments and limit the movement and displacement of brain tissue. The *falx cerebri* is a vertical, large, fibrous tissue, partition of dura, largely separating the two cerebral hemispheres (the right and left upper halves of the brain). The *tentorium cerebelli*, upon which rests the occipital lobes of the cerebrum, is a horizontal fold of dura dividing the posterior portion of the cranial cavity into the upper (supratentorial) compartment and the lower (subtentorial) compartment. These dural folds are seen in figure 37. (There are two more folds, the *falx cerebelli* and the *diaphragma sellae* that do not have great biomechanical importance and are not shown or discussed here; they are only mentioned to recognize their existence.)

The diagram also shows a hole in the horizontal tentorium cerebelli through which passes the midbrain. When there is a disparity in pressure above the tentorium relative to the tissue below the tentorium, such as may occur from cerebral bleeding or swelling, a variety of bad things may occur, ranging from compression of the third cranial nerve (CN3), with resultant third nerve palsy (i.e., a fixed and dilated pupil), to herniation of the cerebellar tonsils causing compression of the vital respiratory and cardiovascular centers in the medulla and, very likely, death therefrom.

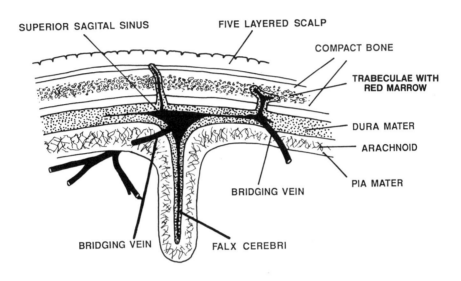

Figure 38
DURAL SINUSES, THE BRIDGING VEINS AND SUBDURAL HEMATOMAS

In this coronal section view of the scalp, the skull, and the meninges, we can see venous blood vessels that are extensions of a dural fold sinus (a venous drainage vessel surrounded by dura mater). These veins reach from the lower scalp, the bony calverium and from the brain substance itself, to drain into the venous dural sinus and thence on to the internal jugular vein and the general circulation.

The veins returning blood from the cerebral cortex to the sinus are termed and labelled ''bridging veins.''

Because they bridge the space from the brain to the dural sinuses, bridging veins are the most easily torn of any of the intracranial blood vessels as they respond to differences of relative motion between the skull and its contents, as in non-contact injuries of the head. In short, **tears of the bridging veins are the most common source of the most common intracranial mass lesion, the *subdural hematoma*.**

- **CN12** — the *hypoglossal* nerve, which literally means "below the tongue," in fact provides pure motor fibers to move the tongue.

While this recitation of the functions of the cranial nerves may be tedious at best, I think it is useful, relatively brief (at least as compared to anatomy texts), and absolutely necessary, for injury to cranial nerves is significant: **about one-third of all closed head injuries have some cranial nerve palsy (i.e., paralysis) and, in over 10 percent of all closed head injuries, cranial nerve palsy is the only neurologic aftermath**[19].

Having now determined that what we see, smell, taste, hear, maintain our balance with, alter blood pressure and heart rate with, secrete tears, saliva and digestive juices with and "a whole lot more" is dependent upon intact cranial nerves, you may be as bewildered as I was to find that destruction of a cranial nerve counts as "Abbreviated Injury Scale" 2, (AIS 2), which AIS defines as a "moderate injury[20];" not even an AIS 3, which is termed as "serious." Tell that to the functionally blinded or deafened; tell them that their injury is not "serious."

The Brain

The brain is a gelatinous organ that weighs about 3 pounds. If removed from the skull and placed on a flat surface, it is deformed and distorted by its own weight. To prevent this resting deformation from happening inside the skull the brain is surrounded by and, in a sense, is floating in, cerebrospinal fluid, resting its most massive portion, the cerebrum, partially upon the anterior floor of the skull and partially upon a fibrous plate (the tentorium cerebelli). Please see figures 37, 38, which show that the two halves of the brain are held vertically separate and have their lateral motion limited by fibrous membranes, the sickle-shaped falx cerebri and falx cerebelli, these dense plates sharing their origins with the tentorium cerebelli.

So that we may understand how the brain is injured by a non-penetrating impact, a "closed head injury" ("CHI" in the literature on the subject), we must first look at the membranes that surround and support the brain and provide it with a portion of its blood supply, which, in turn, means an illustration or two; again please see figures 37 and 38.

The membranes that invest the brain, termed "the meninges," are 3 in number. From the outside inward, they are the dura mater, the arachnoid and the pia mater. They translate roughly as the "strong (or hard) mother," the "spider-like" and the "little mother," respectively, which doesn't at all come across as elegant terminology, even for ancient Latin anatomists.

The outer layer (the dura mater) is a dense fibrous tissue and the thickest of the three membranes. It is adherent to the inner table of the calverium (skull) and serves as both the provider of the blood and nerve supply to the inner table of the skull bones, (i.e., as the periosteal layer of that bone), and as the outer layer of the brain's membranes. Then, in a manner unique within the body, the dura mater splits itself to form meridianly and equatorially aligned venous sinuses, which are fed venous blood from the diploic veins of the bony calverium and from bridging veins from the brain itself. See figure 38, for *it is from tearing these veins that "epidural" hemorrhages (torn diploic veins) and "subdural" and "subarachnoid" hemorrhages (torn bridging veins) originate.* As mentioned previously, it is the dura mater's extensions of the venous sinuses that form the falx cerebri, falx cerebelli and the tentorium cerebelli. Look again at figures 37 and 38.

Categories of Head Injury

This categorization is a simplified classification derived largely from reference[4], with some elements from ref.[7], but it or something close to it is now common throughout head injury literature. Because this book is concerned with the mechanisms of injuries, this version of head injury classification emphasizes mechanisms of injury.

Contact injuries of the head require a blow to the head, but subsequent motion of the head, if present, is not specifically related to the injuries, which *are caused by skull deformation*:

- local deformations (near site of blow) —
  - skull fracture
  - extradural hematoma
  - coup contusion

- distant deformations (far from blow site) —
  - distant vault and basilar fractures

- traveling wave ("shock wave") injuries —
  - contracoup contusion
  - intracerebral bleed/hematoma

Non-contact or acceleration injuries of the head require motion of the head but do not require that the head strikes anything or that anything strikes the head. These injuries will occur only if the head is *accelerated*. Angular acceleration appears to be more causal than linear acceleration and side to side motion appears to be more causal than front to back or back to front motion.

The injuries due to motion of the head rather than to direct blow to the head are from strains (i.e., deformation of tissues from external force loading). The strains may be:

- Surface strains, which cause:
  - subdural hematoma
  - contracoup contusion
  - "intermediate" coup contusion
- Deep strains, which cause:
  - concussion syndromes
  - diffuse axonal injury

According to Gennarelli[4], diffuse axonal injuries (listed above), "are associated with widespread brain damage . . . account for approximately 40 percent of hospitalized head injured patients, for 1/3rd of the deaths and are the most serious cause of persisting neurological disability in survivors." **Almost all DAI results from vehicular crash, which has relatively long duration accelerations, in contrast to accidental falls and assaults, which have impact more brief than crashes and therefore are more commonly associated with sub-dural hematomas.**

To in part summarize closed head injuries: we have listed above what may otherwise be termed:

1) local (or focal/multi-focal) contusions of the brain substance,
2) diffuse injuries of the brain substance (DAI), and
3) bleeding around the brain's coverings (extra-, intra-, and sub-dural bleeding).

Two terms common to head injuries that should be defined are *concussion* and *coma*. They represent a continuum of head injury responses ranging from brief confusion (mild concussion) to profound unresponsiveness (coma) lasting for time periods up to months or even years.

concussion — may be defined as brief unconsciousness, usually lasting only seconds, usually following head impact although there are other causes, such as electrical shock. An important element of concussion relates to its reversibility; the absence of any detectable damage to the brain. The transient loss of consciousness is believed to result from derangements of the electrical activity of the brain. Concussion does not *require* unconsciousness. Confusion, repetitive questions and antegrade or retrograde amnesia are typical indicators of what we term concussion.

coma — may be defined as unconsciousness differing from sleep in that the comatose individual does not respond to stimulation (sound, touch, pain, full bladder, and so forth) while the sleeping individual awakens in response to such stimulation. In addition to head injury, coma may be in response to poisons, brain tumors, deficient cerebral blood flow and many other reasons as well.

There are a variety of quite disturbing and disruptive symptoms that may occur even after quite mild head injuries. These symptoms may include memory, vision, anxiety states, sleep disorders and other psychic and somatic disorders.

Sometimes termed the "post-concussion syndrome," it has been well-demonstrated that cognitive, somatic and emotional symptoms may follow even apparently trivial concussion. In the absence of preexisting neuropsychiatric disorders these complaints usually resolve within 3 months[21].

For the more severe and permanent brain injuries, whatever numbers are provided as human impact tolerance for the brain intact within the body generally are educated guesses, numbers derived from scaling factors converting injury thresholds for primates to human thresholds. But don't for a moment believe that better information doesn't exist because we have not studied head impact tolerance. The 1983 publication "Impact Injury of the Head and Spine," for example[22], is a good summary of the state-of-the-art up to that time, much of it derived from human volunteer tests. Most of what I've seen since then has been an upsurge of mathematical modeling using our increasingly available computer capabilities, in particular wringing out analyses and simulations. Given the scarcely analyzed data banks of human volunteer head and neck impact tests conducted at such locations as the Naval Biodynamics Laboratory in New Orleans, I would be happier if the numerous models seeked comparison with these data banks for at least a first order of validation of the proposed models.

But for the moment, that's all that we have, unless we do as NHTSA did, and, letting expediency govern, use skull fracture data to predict when brain tissue and blood vessels are damaged, while knowing full well that skull fracture bears no predictable relationship to acceleration damage in other tissues, such as brain and blood vessels.

Injuries of the brain are much worsened by reducing blood flow to the brain (as in hemorrhagic or other shock) and by decreased oxygenation of the blood, (as in contused lungs). The pathologic changes caused by decreased cerebral blood flow and decreased cerebral oxygenation are referred to as "hypoxic-ischemic injury." The detailed injury patterns attributable to hypoxic-ischemic damage are beyond the scope of this brief review. Hypoxic-ischemic injury is mentioned here to only to emphasize that it is both characteristic in its injury pattern and that it may be preventable.

In a paper about "patients that talk and die," Rose et al[23] found that more than half of head injury deaths had preventable factors that contributed to the deaths, primarily delay in treatment, inadequate oxygenation and inadequate treatment of shock.

The phrase "patients that talk and die" is a vivid way of stating that, immediately post-injury, the patients were without evidence of contusion or laceration of brain tissue proper; i.e., they could talk (lucidly). That the patients then went on to lose consciousness and then die, generally within but a few hours, is presumptive evidence that there was intracranial bleeding or swelling that was neither diagnosed nor treated adequately or in sufficient time.

By terrible coincidence, two of the several cases sent to me this month for review and analysis involved patients that talked and died. Both patients died before any operative procedure had begun; in both cases they were brought to small hospitals; both cases had 2 or more hours delay, waiting in emergency and radiology departments. At autopsy both cases showed subdural hemorrhages, the smaller being 350 milliliters (about 11 "shot glasses").

Were they waiting in the emergency departments for the neurosurgeon to come to the hospital while the patients were rather obviously busy intracranially bleeding? Were there no immediately available general surgeons who could put in four burr holes? Were the emergency room physicians not trained in emergency procedures such as placing burr holes?

These were 2 cases in the month that this chapter was written, but "patients who talk and die" are a deplorably common avoidable tragedy.

THE EVALUATION OF BRAIN INJURY AND THE PREDICTION OF FUTURE DISABILITY

Although there have been many injury scales developed to assess neurologic injury and predict future neurologic outcomes, Jennett and his coworkers at the University of Glasgow and the Institute of Neurological Sciences, in Glasgow, Scotland, have together given us the tools by which head injuries are now almost universally assessed.

The Glasgow Coma Scale (GCS)[24] is used to assess a patient's condition when first seen by medical or para-medical personnel, so that subsequent serial evaluations using this scale will indicate deterioration or improvement. It does so by a numerical scale derived from eye opening, eye movements, best motor (movements) response and best verbal response. The particular value of the GCS derives from the fact that even multiple assessments by different observers at different times will reliably indicate changes in a patient's neurologic status.

The Glasgow Outcome Scale[19] was developed later, after the Glasgow Coma Scale. The Outcome Scale utilizes 4 possible outcomes after head injury, ranging from "good recovery" to "vegetative state." Good agreement between different observers and studies of outcomes over 1 year from head injury have shown that, of those conscious 3 months after injury and evaluated for at least 18 months, 95 percent reached their maximum improvement category by 12 months[19] post-injury. Head injury outcome information should be important to people in rehabilitation, insurance, and law, and could also be profitably understood by engineers involved in vehicle safety.

The descending order of neurologic deficits following severe closed head injury is:

1) cerebral hemisphere dysfunction (about 60 percent)
2) cranial nerves palsy (about 30 percent)
   (optic nerve 13 percent of all survivors, 9 percent had injury to eye muscle nerves, 8 percent had sensorineural deafness)
3) epilepsy (about 15 percent)
4) no apparent sequelae (about 25 percent)

The above data were derived from a data bank with over 1,000 severely head injured patients, selected as having either a minimum of 6 hours of coma or post-traumatic amnesia of at least 2 days; about 50 percent of those so injured and so selected died.

SUMMARY

Crash injuries of the head are both the leading cause of death in crashes and usually the most common crash injury.

Dividing the head into skull, face and brain, and then sub-dividing injuries of the brain into injuries of the brain and its cranial nerves, we have briefly reviewed these areas while emphasizing a few broad principles. Hopefully, we all recognize that large books and small libraries have been written about injuries to each of these areas or to portions of these areas, and that this book is, after all, a primer.

Looking at bony tolerances we found that the face breaks a lot more readily than the skull. We also noted that facial fractures are complex, disabling, and that facial fractures may also place sensory organs, cranial nerves, and the brain itself in jeopardy.

Skull fractures were found to be related to the skull's anatomy with regard to both their propagation and their potential for mischief, the latter being primarily from associated blood vessel and cranial nerve damage.

Cranial nerve damage was a frequent associate of brain damage, occurring too as the sole residual disability in about 10 percent of all closed head injuries.

We then discussed the brain from the viewpoint of its suspension within its housing, the skull, noting that the brain floats in a thin film of formed fluid, the cerebrospinal fluid, and is both supported and restrained by the larger extensions of its most dense fibrous envelope (dura mater), viz., the falx cerebri, the falx cerebelli, and the tentorium. We also noted that this fibrous envelope is penetrated by blood vessels which bridge the meninges and may be torn by stretching or shear, causing bleeding within the closed volume of the skull. Brain damage or death are the predictable probable outcomes of space-occupying hemorrhages if they are not promptly evacuated.

Brain tissue damage was differentiated into contact and non-contact injuries to emphasize that such injuries as are caused either by *skull deformation* — which requires that something strikes and deforms the bony skull or that the skull is deformed by striking something — or by *acceleration forces*, which deform the brain tissue itself rather than its surrounding skull, thereby directly damaging the brain substance by "strains" and resultant shearing injuries.

Of course, most vehicular crash closed injuries of the head involve both non-contact and contact events. Either type injury may be the dominant injury, although elements of both types are usually present.

Deliberately, there was no specific cataloging or further explanation of the various brain injuries, other than defining concussion and coma, partly because they are the province of the neurosurgeon and partly because they have no clear use to anyone else.

We closed this chapter with an introduction to the Glasgow Coma Scale (GCS) and the Glasgow Outcome Scale (GOS). The GCS is almost universally employed to initially assess and subsequently follow head injuries.

For those among you who may have (non-medical) need to predict the outcome of a closed head injury early after the injury occurs, say an insurance adjuster or a personal injury attorney, the Glasgow Scales should be of considerable use.

BIBLIOGRAPHY

1. Tonge, J.I., O'Reilly, M.J.J., Davison, A. and Johnston, N.G.: Traffic crash fatalities: injury patterns and other factors. *Med J Aust 2*:5, 1972.
2. Hossack, D.W.: The pattern of injuries received by 500 drivers and passengers killed in road accidents. *Med J Aust 2*:193, 1972.
3. Dalmotas, D.J.: Mechanisms of injury to vehicle occupants restrained by three-point seat belts. *SAE* paper 801311, 1980.
4. Gennarelli, T.A.: Head injury biomechanics: A review. *In Head Injury Mechanisms,* AAAM Symposium Report, New Orleans, 1987.
5. Adams, J.H., Graham, D.I. and Gennarelli, T.A.: Contemporary neuropathological considerations regarding brain damage in head injury. In: Becker, D.P., and Povlishock, J.T. (Eds.) *Central Nervous System Trauma Status Report.* NINCDS, NIH, Washington, D.C., 1985.
6. Papo, I., Caruselli, G., Scarpelli, M. and Luongo, A.: Mass lesions of the frontal lobes in acute head injuries: a comparison with temporal lesions. *Acta Neurochir 62*:47, 1982.
7. Salazar, A.M.: Neurologic sequelae of closed and penetrating head injury. Recent Advances in Head Injury. Course #106, *Am Acad Neurol,* April 1988.
8. Moritz, A.R.: Mechanical injuries of the skeletomuscular system. In *The Pathology of Trauma*, 2nd ed. Lea & Feabiger, Philadelphia, 1954.
9. Harvey, F.H. and A.M. Jones: "Typical" basal skull fracture of both petrous bones: an unreliable indicator of head impact site. *J Forensic Sci, 25*:280, 1980.
10. Lissner, H.R. and E.S. Gurdjian: Experimental cerebral concussion. *ASME 60-WA-273*, 1960.
11. Ono, K., Kikuchi, A., Nakamura, M., Kobayashi, H. and N. Nakamura: Human head tolerance to sagittal impact reliable estimation deduced from experimental head injury using subhuman primates and human cadaver skulls. *SAE* paper 801303, 1980.
12. Vance, B.M.: Fractures of the skull. *Arch Surg, 14*:1023, 1927.
13. Gurdjian, E.S., Webster, J.E. and H.R. Lissner: Observations on prediction of fracture site in head injury. *Radiology, 60*:226, 1953.
14. Huelke, D.F., Smock, W.S., Fuller, P.F. and G.R. Nichols: Basilar skull fractures produced by facial impacts — case histories and a review of the literature. *SAE* paper 881711, 1988.

15. Voigt, G.E. and G. Skold: Ring fractures of the base of the skull. *J Trauma, 14*:494, 1974.
16. Human tolerance to impact conditions as related to motor vehicle design. *SAE* J885, rev. July 1986.
17. Zeidler, F., Pletschen, B., Mattern, B., Alt, B., Miksch, T., Eichendorf, W. and S. Reiss: Development of a new injury cost scale. *AAAM 33rd Ann Proc,* p. 231, 1989.
18. Grimm, R.J., Hemenway, W.G., Lebray, P.R. and F.O. Black: The perilymph fistula syndrome defined in mild head trauma. *Acta Oto-Laryngol Suppl 464*:1, 1989.
19. Jennett, B., Snock, J., Bond, M. and N. Brooks: Disability after severe head injury: observations on the use of the Glasgow outcome scale. *J Neurol Neurosurg Psychiatry 44*:285, 1981.
20. Abbreviated injury scale 1985 revision. Arlington, *AAAM*, 1985.
21. Levin, H.S., Mattis, S., Ruff, R.M., Eisenberg, H.M., Marshall, L.F., Tabbador, K., High, W.M. and R.F. Frankowski: Neurobehavioral outcome following minor head injury: a three-center study. *J Neurosurg 66*:234. 1987.
22. Ewing, C.L., Thomas, D.J., Sances, Jr., A. and S.J. Larson (Eds.): *Impact injury of the head and spine*, Thomas, Springfield, 1983.
23. Rose, J., Valtonen, S. and B. Jennett: Avoidable factors contributing to death after head injury. *BMJ 2*:615, 1977.
24. Teasdale, G. and B. Jennett: Assessment of coma and impaired consciousness: A practical scale. *Lancet 81*, 1974.

CHAPTER 9

THE SPINE

GENERAL

When we say "the spine" we speak of an anatomic unit divisible into 2 entirely unrelated structures and functions: the musculoskeletal spine and the spinal cord that it contains.

The Importance and Vulnerability of the Spine

Between one-half and four-fifths of the working population of the United States will have memorable low back pain at some time during their working years. About one-quarter of the adult population will have low back pain at some time *this very year* (i.e., within any given year)[1]. To put some numbers with this statement, we are saying that about 40 million adults will have low back pain this year. And that's only low back pain, which is lumbar or lumbo-sacral pain; I could not find reliable information for the prevalence and incidence of cervical and thoracic back pain.

Figures from the Insurance Institute for Highway Safety suggest that at least 4.5 million motor vehicle injuries occur annually, of which some 85 percent are minor injuries. Putting these figures together, it may be said that *in any given 12 month period, about 1 of every 12 adults with minor injury from an auto accident will also be expected to have low back pain whose cause is unrelated to their auto accident.*

I have included in this chapter general information about degenerative disease of the musculoskeletal spine (including its intervertebral discs) in order to explain how this may be so.

Low back pain may have its origin in the musculoskeletal system, in regional nerve involvement, or the pain may be referred from other areas of the body. But "most pain and disability of the low back (lumbosacral spine) is mechanical in nature[2]."

The most devastating disability from spinal injury is reserved for damage to the spinal cord itself, that bundle of nerve fibers running downward from the brain to

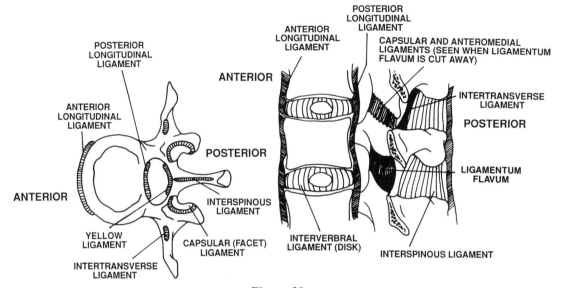

Figure 39
**LUMBAR VERTEBRAE AND THE LIGAMENTS THAT JOIN THEM TOGETHER,
ESPECIALLY THE INTERVERTEBRAL DISC**

Seen here are lumbar vertebrae, in plan view (to the left) and in side view (to the right, with a portion of the bodies of the vertebrae and the neural archway closest to the reader removed for clarity of certain relationships).

Nine ligaments are shown here as connections between any 2 vertebrae. The left illustration shows 8 of them clearly, to which should be added an intervertebral disc.

Note that, except for the intervertebral disc, all other intervertebral ligaments are linearly aligned and therefore resist *tension*, although they are put into tension by such other motions between vertebrae as rotation, flexion (in any direction) and shear. They are neither stressed nor strained by compression. Note too that, of all the intervertebral ligaments, only the intervertebral disc has a liquid center.

Those of you who play golf probably know that a golf ball is made of circumferential fibers wrapped around a liquid center, much like an intervertebral disc. Why then does the intervertebral disc have a liquid center? Blaise Pascal would say it is because of Pascal's Principle, which noted that pressure in a liquid is everywhere the same. Thus when the column of vertebral bodies is compressed (and *all* of the other ligaments between vertebrae are therefore relaxed), *only* the intervertebral disc is effected by compression. Because of its liquid center (and Pascal's Principle) the compressive pressure is distributed not only upwards and downwards, but also to the encircling thickest portion of the intervertebral disc, thus reducing the load-per-unit-area to all portions of the disc.

Consider that every step we take, every time we sit, every time we lift anything at all, we axially compress the intervertebral disc. As the sole ligamentous defender of the spinal column in compression, the intervertebral disc needs all of the mechanical design help that it can get.

When two vertebrae are moved in any direction other than compression, the other ligaments are put into stretch (tension). Where we have data for flexion, extension, rotation and shear, in vertebral units with *all* ligaments intact, the ligaments other than the intervertebral disc will tear before the disc will. While it is true that the intervertebral disc is somewhat compressed by motions other than axial compression, it cannot be highly stressed in these other motions in the absence of concurrent axial compression.

connect with sensors, muscles, and glandular tissues throughout the entire body. Despite our modern medical armamentarium, injury to the spinal cord is still largely untreatable and unrepairable. Spinal cord injuries to occupants of crashed cars appear to represent about 40 to 50 percent of all fatal and non-fatal spinal cord injuries of any cause[3]. That's half of about 10,000 new cases of acute spinal cord injury that occur annually[4]. We will later see why, of all possible locations, the first two cervical vertebrae are uniquely vulnerable places for damage to either the bony spine or the spinal cord. Pedestrians, cyclists and motor vehicle occupants appear to have the greatest frequency of such injuries[3].

In the spine, in contrast with other regions of the body, the most common injuries frequently are serious injuries and often are the causes of permanent impairment.

AN OVERVIEW OF THE ANATOMY OF THE SPINE

The spine serves as the axial skeleton's main load-bearing member for the midsection of the body or trunk (as was shown back in chapter 4, when we put together a load-bearing skeleton). Cylinders of bone are stacked upon each other and bound together by 3 ligaments between each pair of cylinders (the anterior and posterior longitudinal ligaments and an intervertebral body annular ligamentous disc). See figure 39.

As they go footward, each bony cylinder is slightly larger than the one above it, because each cylinder must carry successively greater portions of the body's weight, and, by being larger, the load upon each square inch of cylinder surface does not increase as much as it would if all vertebral bodies were of the same size.

In addition to its load-bearing skeletal function the spine also provides a bony shield to protect the spinal cord and nerves connecting to the spinal cord. Each cylinder of bone has an arch of bone (the neural arch) on its back side (posterior surface) which largely surrounds the spinal cord. Figure 39 shows a typical lumbar vertebra from the stacked column of bony cylinders and their posterior neural arches, the term "vertebra" being the name applied to each of the segmental units, the cylinder of bone, its neural arch, facet joints (discussed below) and 3 bony appendages for the connection of muscles and ligaments, the spinous process and two transverse processes. According to how you wish to dissect them, what spinal level you are dealing with, or how you wish to tally them, there are a total of 7 to 12 rather substantial ligaments that bind together the vertebral bodies, arches, facets and processes of any 2 vertebrae. The numerous ligaments, muscles and joints provide for the third func-

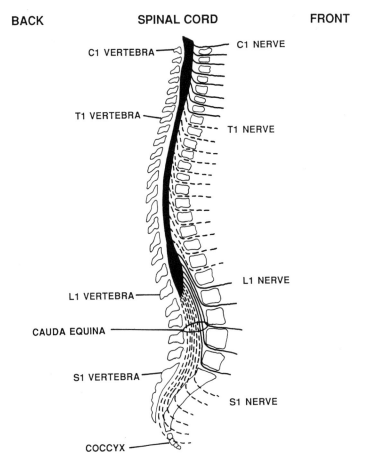

BACK **SPINAL CORD** **FRONT**

C1 VERTEBRA — C1 NERVE

T1 VERTEBRA — T1 NERVE

L1 NERVE

L1 VERTEBRA

CAUDA EQUINA

S1 VERTEBRA

S1 NERVE

COCCYX

Figure 40
THE RELATIONSHIP BETWEEN THE SPINAL CORD AND THE FORAMINA
THROUGH WHICH THE SPINAL NERVES EMERGE

This view is a vertical slice through the middle of the spine and the spinal cord (i.e., through the median plane). Note that:

1)   only at C1 do the nerves emerge at about the same level that there are appropriate foramina for them to emerge through;

2)   the spinal cord ends at about L1/L2;

3)   there are 2 dilatations of the spinal cord, the first from about C2 to about C6 (spinal segments C4 to T1), the second from about T11 to L2 (spinal segments L2 to S3). The upper dilatation accommodates the extra innervation of the brachial plexus for the upper limbs; the lower dilatation accommodates the innervation for the lumbar and sacral plexuses supplying the lower limbs;

4)   because the bony spine has grown so much more than did the spinal cord, the lower lumbar and sacral nerves emerge from the bony spine a very great distance from where they first emerged from the spinal cord itself.

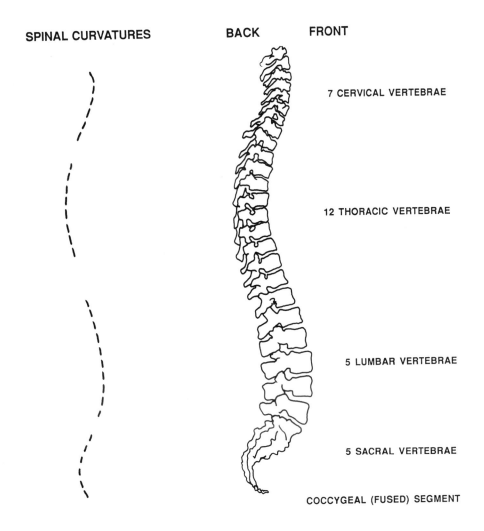

SPINAL CURVATURES   BACK   FRONT

7 CERVICAL VERTEBRAE

12 THORACIC VERTEBRAE

5 LUMBAR VERTEBRAE

5 SACRAL VERTEBRAE

COCCYGEAL (FUSED) SEGMENT

Figure 41
FOUR GROUPS OF VERTEBRAE AND THEIR CURVATURES

This simple drawing identifies the grouping of vertebrae into 7 cervical, 12 thoracic, 5 lumbar and 5 sacral (fused) vertebrae, with the somewhat vestigial four or so coccygeal vertebrae located at the very bottom of the vertebral column, as a forward facing projection.

The serpentine curvatures reverse at each group of vertebrae. As viewed from in back of the individual, we see a cervical concavity, a thoracic convexity, a lumbar concavity and a sacral convexity. These charming curves are readily deformable into the poor postures we often see.

The cervical and lumbar curvatures are considered to be secondary curves in that they do not develop until we stand up and walk.

tion of the spine, that of allowing flexibility and mobility while concurrently providing the spine's other 2 functions, that of bearing the skeletal load and that of protecting the spinal cord and its connecting nerves.

The *spinal cord* is a bundle of fiber tracts extending from the brain to about the L2 level, ultimately connecting through nerve branches with sensors, muscles, and glands throughout the all of the body except the head. The spinal cord weighs but 1.5 ozs., or about a thirtieth as much as the brain itself. As with the brain, the cord is invested by the same 3 meningeal coverings. It is about an inch in diameter and merely 16 to 18 inches long. Only two thirds of the adult spinal canal contains the cord.

To orient you topographically, the cord ends at a level (L1, L2) a few inches *above* the umbilicus. It is only in the 24th week of gestation that the fetal spinal canal is filled by the spinal cord. By birth only 3 quarters of the length of the spinal canal is occupied by the spinal cord, which ends at about the level of the third lumbar vertebra. Thereafter the bony vertebral case grows at a rate slightly faster than the spinal cord, so that by maturity, the vertebral column is so much longer than the spinal cord that its sacral nerves must extend a great distance before they can emerge. To put it otherwise, only at C7 and above do the nerves attach to the spinal cord near the same level as they emerge from the vertebral column; below C7 the nerve roots attach to the spinal cord at successively greater distances from the intervertebral foramens through which they must finally leave the bony spine. This is difficult to say but is easily seen in figure 40.

The bony spine is a flexible, segmented, loadbearing conduit for the spinal cord and its segmental offshoots (nerves). It has 33 bony segments (vertebrae), categorized into 5 groups, from the head downward, termed cervical, thoracic, lumbar, sacral and coccygeal vertebrae, the groups of vertebrae having 7, 12, 5, 5 and 4 segments, respectively. The lowest 4 vertebrae generally fuse into a single bone, the coccyx, and the 5 segments above (superior to) the coccyx also fuse into a single bone, called the sacrum. See figure 41, which also shows each of the vertebral groupings and how each group's curvature is the reverse of the one above it.

Each of the groups of vertebrae are different from the other and within each group the vertebrae may also be quite different. For example, the first two cervical vertebrae, the atlas and the axis, are completely unlike each other and unlike any other vertebrae.

The first cervical vertebra, the atlas, articulates with and supports thereby the occipital condyles of the base of the skull, allowing for "moderate" flexion and extension of the head on the neck, but virtually no axial rotation[5]. It is composed only of an anterior and a posterior bony arch, lacking the cylindrical anterior body present in all other vertebrae (except the axis). The second cervical vertebra (the axis) also lacks an apparent body and it too is composed of 2 arches, the posterior arch providing a distinctive, large, upward extension, somewhat resembling a good-sized canine tooth and named therefore the "dens," which, with its articulation with the posterior arch of the atlas, provides the pivot about which the head may be axially rotated an "extensive" amount while permitting only limited flexion and extension[5].

The remaining cervical vertebrae have distinctive lateral wedges on the superior lateral surfaces of their vertebral bodies, termed the uncinate (hook-like) processes, which apparently exist to limit lateral flexion and are present only in the neck. Finally, the first 6 cervical vertebrae are also remarkable in that they partly house a pair of arteries, the vertebral arteries, within (C1) and against their bony neural arch structures (C2-7). The vertebral arteries later merge within the cranium to form the basilar artery, providing the chief blood supply to the posterior portion of the brain. Note here then that vertebral arteries have little to do with vertebrae except to travel with and within them and have everything to do with the blood supply of the posterior brain. Comminuted fractures of the neural arches of the cervical vertebrae, particularly C1, where the arteries pass through holes within the bony structure of C1, have the potency to injure or tear the vertebral arteries, and therefore some cervical fractures have the potency to seriously compromise blood supply to the brain itself. Tears of the vertebral arteries are often fatal.

Traveling downward from the 7 cervical vertebrae, the next 12 vertebrae are called thoracic or dorsal vertebrae. Thoracic, which refers to the chest, seems a better term than dorsal, since each of the thoracic vertebrae are distinguishable from other vertebrae by 1 or 2 indentations on the posterior centrum (body) and on the transverse processes where the ribs articulate (form joints) with the vertebrae. As you might expect, having the 12 thoracic vertebrae effectively tied to the rib cage and its musculature considerably modifies and limits the mobility of this segment of the spine.

Below the rib cage are 5 lumbar vertebrae, easily distinguished from other vertebrae by their relative massiveness, necessary to support the weight of all of the body above their level. In addition to their size and absence of facets and demifacets to articulate with ribs, the lumbar vertebrae differ from the thoracic vertebrae just above them by an abrupt change in the angle of the facet joints (discussed below), the thoracic facets facing mostly forward or rearward and the lumbar facets being axially rotated almost 90 degrees, facing primarily either laterally or medially. Thus injury to the thoracolumbar spine (especially T11, T12, L1 and L2) may often be attributable to the abrupt change in stiffness from the thoracic to the lumbar spine[5].

As noted above, the sacral and coccygeal vertebrae are fused together in the 2 groups, although there often is some limited movement between the first and second coccy-

CERVICAL EXTENSION AND FLEXION

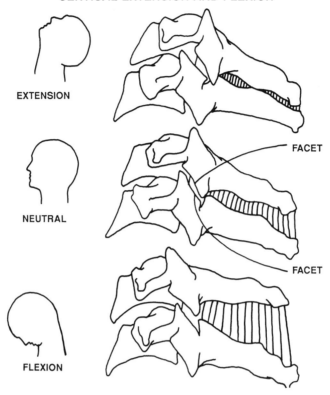

Figure 42
FACET JOINTS AND THEIR RELATIVE MOTION WITH FLEXION AND EXTENSION, SHOWN HERE FOR LOWER CERVICAL VERTEBRAE (after ref.⁵)

Note the relationship between the articular surfaces of the facets as they move from flexion to extension. The intervertebral spaces mirror the wedging of the facets.

In flexion, because the upper vertebral body tilts forward with respect to the underlying vertebral body, the anterior superior surface of the inferior facet appears to gauge the articular surface of the superior facet. (Is this how osteoarthritis starts in the lower cervical vertebrae?) Extension appears less potentially damaging to the articular surfaces of inferior facets than does flexion.

Extension is here limited by bony contact between the posterior neural arches and the spinous processes as well as by tension in the anterior longitudinal ligament and in the anterior portion of the annulus of the disc.

Flexion is limited by tension in several ligaments, including: the posterior cervical ligament (the interspinous ligament), the ligamentous capsules of the facet joints, the ligamentum nuchae and the ligamenta flava, the posterior longitudinal ligament and, of course, the posterior portion of the intervertebral disc.

Please take note that extension drives the nucleus pulposus forward (anteriorly), which makes claims of posterior herniation of a cervical disc improbable, to say the least, as a result of a rear impact! Flexion will, of course, do just the opposite to the nucleus, moving the nucleus pulposus rearward (posteriorly).

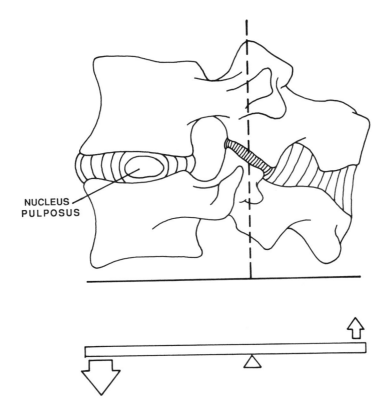

NUCLEUS
PULPOSUS

Figure 43
LUMBAR VERTERAE
THEIR AXIS OF ROTATION IN FLEXION

This drawing shows the fulcrum for lumbar flexion occurring at about the facet joints, thus providing what the physicists refer to as a "first order lever system" but which we could as easily identify as a teeter-board or teeter-totter board, according to where we were raised. This is shown too in refs.[5] [7] with about the same fulcrum location.

Lower lumbar vertebrae carry more body weight than any other vertebrae. They often suffer greater wear and tear and have the highest incidence of disc herniation than any of the vertebrae. They also have the greatest flexibility in flexion of any vertebral group and are flexed more in association with lifting, I would expect, than any other vertebrae. As pointed out by Kapandji[7], the lever system illustrated here shows *direct, passive absorption of compression by the intervertebral disc and shows both indirect and active resistance to flexion by the paravertebral muscles.*

geal vertebrae and occasionally there may be some (minimal) motion between all or any of the coccygeal segments.

With the exception of the first 2 cervical vertebrae, and the sacrum and coccyx as well, the frontal (anterior) loadbearing portion of each segment (vertebra) is a cylinder of cancellous bone which, you will remember, is bone containing red marrow and having the biomechanical virtue of absorbing considerable energy as it is crushed. In addition to the intervertebral disc joint (*a symphysis joint*) between each cylinder of bone (the vertebral bodies) there is an important second pair of joints between each pair of vertebrae, termed the *facet joints* (see figure 42).

There are 4 facet surfaces per vertebra, which form 2 facet joints between any 2 vertebrae. Facet joints are true *synovial joints*, comprised of a fibrous capsule, synovial membrane and articular cartilage, much as in say, a knuckle joint. As true synovial joints, the facets are subject to all of the degenerative wear-and-tear (osteo-arthritic) changes common to diarthroidal synovial joints, and we will discuss these changes shortly, for they are an important source of back pain.

The facets represent additional load-bearing surfaces, additional joints helping the vertebral bodies to carry the weight of the person's body above any given vertebral level. There is indirect evidence that about one-fifth of total compressive loading of the spine is borne by the facets and about four-fifths is borne by the intervertebral disc joints[6]. The contributions of the facets and their capsules are more complex for other motions, such as torsion and tension[5].

The facet joints also serve as fulcrums or pivot points when one vertebra is flexed forward or extended on the one below it (see figure 42). The dimensions of this pivot are such that a mechanical advantage is provided to the posterior ligaments and bony elements, an advantage of about 3:2 as compared to the vertebral bodies (see figure 43). All of which means that when loaded and forced in flexion, the posterior musculoskeletal elements of a pair of vertebrae will have about two-thirds of the load (in tension) that the vertebral bodies will be subject to (in compression). In addition, the anterior vertebral body has about 75 percent of the compressive strength of the posterior portion of a vertebral body[7]. It is small wonder then that vertebral body wedge compression fractures occur so commonly in the absence of detectable damage to the posterior elements.

As noted above, the inclination of the articular surfaces of the facet joints is both different and quite characteristic for each of the groups of vertebrae, the cervical facet angles being most shallow and the lumbar facets being most vertical. This observation gains whatever importance it holds because it is the inclination of these facets that largely determines much of the mobility of any pair of vertebrae. Your observation of yourself and others has already taught you that the neck seems to be more mobile than the lower back, thus you may conclude that the more shallow the facet angle, the more mobile is any particular vertebral pair. You would be correct to so conclude. But you would only be correct for certain motions: that of bending from side to side (i.e., lateral flexion) and for rotation about the long axis of the spine. Lumbar flexion (forward bending) exceeds cervical flexion in range, although cervical extension (rearward bending) exceeds lumbar extension[7].

We have seen that, depending upon what part of the spinal column we are considering, there are 7 to 12 ligaments connecting any 2 vertebrae. (See figure 39.) *The intervertebral disc is just one of these several ligaments.* So let me address those who use the usual anatomic models made to demonstrate intervertebral disc anatomy for purposes of litigation: be warned and aware that such models omit all of the other several intervertebral ligaments and omit all of the surrounding massive musculature that ties vertebra to vertebra. Almost any anatomy text will yield a proper representation of all of the intervertebral ligaments, which may make the "litigation disc model" then appear as the misrepresentation that it really is, although admittedly, it is possible that such omission may be unintentional.

THE INTERVERTEBRAL DISCS

As their name tells us, the intervertebral discs are discoid ligaments that, along with the anterior and posterior intervertebral ligaments, connect together the cylindrical bodies of any two vertebrae. The discs are thinnest in the chest (thoracic) region and thickest in the low back (lumbar) region. They are also thicker in front (anteriorly) than in back (posteriorly) in the neck and low back, thus accounting for the curves in these spinal segments. The thickness of the interverteral discs are a substantial part of one's height, representing about 25 percent of the height (length) of the vertebral column[8].

The intervertebral disc is different from other intervertebral ligaments in two important and related ways: 1) the disc has a centeral gelatinous portion, devoid of blood vessels and nearly 90 percent water, called the "nucleus pulposus" and 2) *the disc, by its central substance, is the only ligament that resists axial compression of the spinal column.*

In 1960 Nachemson reported on studies done in Sweden using young normal human volunteer subjects with a needle-pressure transducer inserted into the nucleus pulposus of their third lumbar vertebrae[6] while the subjects performed simple and common daily maneuvers. This and numerous similar subsequent studies by Nachemson have provided relative information as to what does and what does not cause changes in intradiscal pressures and which maneuver causes greater or lesser intradiscal pressures.

Using the supine position as base, simply standing at rest about doubled the pressure in L3, as did coughing, straining or flexing forward 20 degrees. Flexing forward 40 degrees quadrupled the L3 intradiscal pressure, while flexing forward 20 degrees and rotating 20 degrees while holding 22 pounds in hand increased the intradiscal pressure about 8 times. Lifting 22 pounds with the back flexed or while holding only 12.5 pounds at the end of extended arms also caused nearly an 8 times increase in intradiscal pressure.

Invariably, the greatest intradiscal pressure occurred only when lifting, even when lifting such modest loads as 25 pounds or less. (Twenty five pounds, it may be noted, is about the weight of the average 18 month old male baby. Young mothers, fathers and even elderly grandparents will bend, twist and lift such creatures many times each day, often with great pleasure while doing so, despite the intradiscal pressure threat implicit therein!)

Laboratory studies utilizing cadaveric spinal segments have attempted to herniate the nucleus pulposus. They have shown that, while axial compression by itself does not cause disc herniation[9][10], axial compression is a necessary component of such herniation when combined with bending and/or twisting[11][12][13][14]. Bending, twisting and shear by themselves are severe loads, but do not by themselves seem to cause disc herniation *in the intact human back*. Thus incidents and accidents wherein axial compression of the vertebral column is not present as a significant force are not likely causes of a herniated disc (i.e., a "ruptured disc," or "herniated nucleus pulposus," all of which are the same as the highly popular but misnamed "slipped disc").

Although I have largely avoided presenting controversy before the readers of this primer, it is here unavoidable because of the astonishing volume of litigation relating to herniated discs and the presumed causes of disc herniation. Without going on to write a book about mechanisms of intervertebral disc disease, let us note that hypotheses have been put forth in which single directional loads may cause disc herniation. They are less than persuasive to me, at least partly because they utilize isolated "vertebral units," or a pair of vertebrae denuded of muscles and, varying with the study, are either stripped of some or most intervertebral ligaments or even some bony elements. To me, they are most unnatural models of reality.

Farfan[15], for example, has proposed that torsional loading alone may be the major disc injuring load. In Farfan's study, the average rotational failure was 22.6 degrees, with articular processes failing at an average angle of 12 degrees, interspinous and supraspinous ligaments failing at an average of 12 degrees, and intervertebral discs failing at an average of 16 degrees. Thus if pure torsion does indeed cause common disc failure, we would expect that when there was disc failure we should also expect antecedent failure of both spinous process ligaments and of articular processes.

Of course, that simply doesn't occur in the real world, which then would seem to disallow pure torsion as a cause of common disc failure. And lastly, it is also well known that motions in the intact vertebrae are coupled, which is to say that almost no motion exists in purely a single degree of freedom; except for pure axial compression, all other motions are coupled to some extent.

Again, take note that when the normal vertebral column is subjected only to pure axial compression — that is, when the vertebral bodies are displaced toward each other in the absence of shear, bending or twisting — then the cartilaginous endplates of the vertebral bodies will fracture *before* the intervertebral discs herniate[16][17][18][19].

Epidemiologically, when causal factors are compared to the incidence of the disease, then the real world tells us that torsion coupled with compression and/or flexion coupled with compression are the most probable modes of acute disc failure[13].

The real world also tells us that discs are not suddenly struck with disease; rather, disc failure is an event relatively terminal in a long term disease process requiring many years to evolve.

As to the vernacular "slipped disc" (a misleading but colorful term I still often hear), the misconception or misunderstanding that is generated by this term is beyond my imagination. After all, the intervertebral disc is simply the fibrous portion of a fibrocartilaginous joint. It is neither slimy nor slippery and there isn't any way in the world that it can "slip" anywhere. Try as I may, I cannot conjure up what picture is in the mind of someone speaking of his or her "slipped disc," or what is in the mind of someone who hears this expression. This is not to nit-pick terminology; it is just that I believe that if you cannot understand and visualize what any particular injury consists of, then you also cannot possibly understand what it is, how it occurs, how to treat it and how to perhaps prevent its occurrence.

AGING AND THE SPINE, OR WHAT IS A NORMAL SPINE?

The spine makes us ask "when does an abnormal finding become so frequent an event that what was abnormal becomes the norm?"

By the relatively reliable assays of both myelography[20] and computer-assisted tomography ("CAT scans")[21], **about one-third of *asymptomatic* patients were found to have abnormal lumbar spines, with the diagnoses of herniated disc, facet degeneration and spinal stenosis being the most common.**

Under age 40, 1 of every 5 *asymptomatic* individuals were found to have herniations of lumbar discs[21].

Necessarily, we must ask "What is normal?" when 25 to 35 percent of everyone under age 40 *without back pain* has either a herniated lumbar disc or other apparent radiologic signs of disease.

One-half of the *asymptomatic* forty-and-over age group had "abnormal" CAT scans. I don't know about you, but certainly, when one-half of the asymptomatic population has certain findings and one-half doesn't, I have great difficulty with the idea that either half is normal and the other half isn't.

That a large percentage of the population has back pain without radiologic evidence of trauma or disease and a large percentage of the population has radiologic evidence of disease and has no back pain certainly suggests that when back pain and radiologic evidence of trauma and disease are simultaneously present, we should at least be cautious about these events being causally related. In fact, we should be very cautious.

DEGENERATIVE DISEASE OF THE SPINE

Salter's clear and brief description of degenerative disease of the lumbar spine[22] involves 2 conditions that occur together and represent varying degrees of acceleration of the normal aging process. They are:

1) disc degeneration, and
2) degenerative joint disease of the facet joints (also termed DJD or osteoarthritis).

Disc Degeneration

Disc degeneration must be present for disc herniation to occur but not all degenerative disc disease results in disc herniation.

Early in adult life the discs start aging, desiccating the gelatinous substance of the nucleus pulposus, losing turgor and losing actual disc height as part of the process. This certainly is normal over age 50 and abnormal in say, the 20s. Conversely, herniation or protrusion of the nucleus or annulus occurs in the young adult whose discs still have much turgor, and disc herniation is relatively rare after age 50, when the nucleus is liable to be dry, lumpy and leathery.

The Natural History of Herniation of the Intervertebral Disc

Herniation, or rupture, or prolapse, or protrusion (all near equivalents) of the intervertbral disc are not invariable consequences of disc degeneration, although they are not rare consequences. Most common in young males, the most frequent sites in order of occurrence, are L4-5, L5-S1 and L3-4[22]. The L4-5 and L5-S1 together represent 95 percent of all lumbar disc herniations[1].

Our discussion of disc disease will emphasize lumbar disc pathology but our presentation of crash injury will emphasize injuries to the upper (cervical and thoracic) regions. A detailed presentation of the pathologic process of disc degeneration may be found in Armstrong[23].

Pain is generally the earliest symptom of disc degeneration. Weber[24] found that 90 percent of patients studied showed some 10 years of low back pain preceding the onset of pain radiating down a leg and/or numbness and tingling caused by nerve root compression. A bit more than half of the patients studied recollected a *possible* precipitating event, ranging from abrupt movement to lifting, which is to say that *about 45 percent of the lumbar disc herniations Weber studied could not think of a possible traumatic origin of their pain.* **It may be said that trauma is a precipitating event rather than the cause of disc disease.**

An analysis of the histories of 2504 patients with lumbar disc herniations proven by operations found that low back pain usually preceded the onset of leg pain (radicular pain) by about two years[25].

Typically, the low back pain of the pre-herniation interval (of years) lasts but a few days at a time, and usually gets better by limiting activity and/or by bedrest. As time passes, the intervals between low back pain periods get shorter and both the intensity and the duration of the painful periods get longer.

This intermittent nature of disc disease pain should be considered as a characteristic of the disease process. A pattern of relentless and progressive pain would be more typical of infection or tumor.

Sciatica, or pain along the path of the sciatic nerve and its branches, is not a necessary component of the clinical course of lumbar disc disease. It is not uncommon for a patient with a herniated lumbar disc to never have had sciatica. It is also not uncommon for a patient to have one or more episodes of sciatica for a variety of reasons other than lumbar disc disease or disc herniation.

Segmental Narrowing

With increasing age, narrowing of the disc space due to the lessening volume of the nucleus pulposus permits the discs to bulge, which induces osteophytes to form on adjacent vertebral bodies. This pathology is described as *spondylosis* (and, less commonly, as *spinal osteophytosis*). The most common locations of such bony spurs are C5-7 and L4-S1. "Such osteophytes are detected radiographically in 90 percent of all individuals over the age of 60[22]." Ordinarily, simple bulging of one or more discs causes no problems. However, when there is narrowing of the bony spinal canal or of the intervertebral foramina through which the nerve roots emerge, simple disc bulges *may* then impinge on central canal contents, such as the cauda equina in the lumbar region, or the spinal cord in the neck, or lateral components, such as emerging nerve roots or their blood supply. This narrowing of either the bony spinal canal or of the intervertebral foramina is termed *spinal stenosis* and may be either congenital or a result of degenerative processes in the disc or the facets. Acute mechanical trauma is a most improbable cause of spinal stenosis.

Segmental Instability

Salter[22] considers the changes in the discs (described above) to cause:

1) loss of the smooth motion of the lumbar spinal segments, and
2) excessive motion of these segments.

Excessive segment motion in turn causes and is radiologically marked by so-called "traction spurs," which are small bony outgrowths (osteophytes) arising from the margins of the bodies of the involved adjoining vertebrae.

Segmental Hyperextension

Degeneration of the anterior annular disc fibers also permits excessive segmental hyperextension, which in turn allows persistent lumbar hyperextension. This excessive hyperextension strains the posterior facet joints, allows for their misalignment and "causes degenerative joint disease (osteoarthritis) of these synovial joints with loss of articular cartilage, eburnation of subchondral bone and formation of osteophytes[22]." The posterior facet joints may even subluxate because of the segmental hyperextension.

Clinical Manifestations

Disc degeneration by itself causes neither signs nor symptoms. It is the pathologic changes from segmental instability, segmental hyperextension, segmental narrowing or secondary effects of herniation of the intervertebral disc that have the ability to cause signs and symptoms.

Central stenosis may cause diffuse back pain (and spasm of back muscles) while lateral stenosis may cause radicular pain and dysthesias.

Let me emphasize that all low back pain does not come from pathologic changes in vertebrae or their soft tissues. Lesions of the genitourinary tract, pelvic organs, descending aorta and its branches, infections or tumors of the spinal cord or the cauda equina, and other bony and soft tissue injuries of the pelvis or back muscles — all these and more must be distinguished from vertebral column pain or at least be investigated as possible causes. Mcnab[26] and Weisel[1] are very good sources for further studying, classifying and understanding low back pain; Cailliet[2] has a helpful, heavily illustrated and somewhat simplified presentation of this complex subject.

SPINAL TRAUMA

Injuries of the spine will be divided into:

1) musculoskeletal injuries of the vertebral column, and
2) injuries of the spinal cord.

Vertebral column injuries will be further divided into each of the five groups of vertebrae since each group of vertebrae have their own anatomic and biomechanical peculiarities.

Texts of especial value for understanding spinal trauma include Rothman and Simeone's *The Spine*[27], White and Panjabi's *Clinical Biomechanics of the Spine*[5],

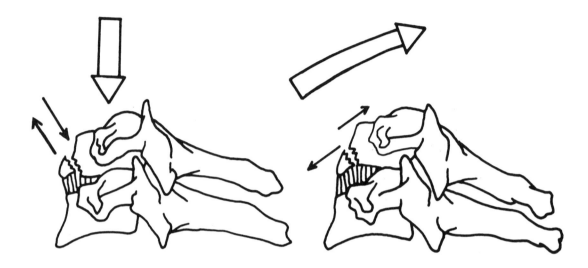

Figure 44
THE TEAR-DROP FRACTURE (after ref.[7])

This fracture, generally of the lower cervical vertebrae, is often associated with serious spinal injury. The term "tear drop" refers to the appearance of a fragment of bone torn from the anterior inferior aspect of the cervical vertebral body. It tells us of a fracture dislocation of the vertebra.

The radiologic appearance does not suggest that two quite different mechanisms may cause this fracture dislocation, nor does the radiologic appearance necessarily even suggest the severe quadriplegia (from an "anterior spinal syndrome") that may accompany this radiologic sign.

This fracture dislocation may be caused *either* by compression (which shears off the bone fragment) *or* by extension, which separates the tear drop fragment from the body by tension (pulling).

The lesson to be learned from all this is that even a so-called classical radiologic appearance cannot tell which mechanism caused it, nor does it necessarily tell the true extent of the injury; it can only indicate the *residual* injury after even severely displaced fragments may have returned to near-normal position.

and Ghista and Frankel's *Spinal Cord Injury Medical Engineering*[28].

Mechanisms of Musculoskeletal Injuries of the Vertebral Column

General

Our interest remains in understanding and, where possible, defining mechanisms of trauma. In reference[28] the problems of inferring causal mechanisms of spinal trauma from x-ray appearances and from residual deformities are particularly well presented and discussed.

Clearly, residual deformity does not tell us what the maximum deformation was at the time of the maximum loading.

The authors of ref.[28] emphasize that **different external loads may produce the same internal motions and therefore the same internal lesion.** For example, the well-known anterior inferior vertebral body lip fracture (figure 44) is generally ascribed to a hyperextension load, but it may also be produced by the exactly opposite loading, that of hyperflexion, if the hyperflexion is accompanied by compression.

In addition, for the same loads, **muscular pretensioning may modify the injury sites and therefore also change the resultant injuries**[29]. It also has been widely noted that **identical injury-site loads may cause a wide variety of injuries, depending upon which of a particular individual's structural elements is the weakest link.**

Based on their years of studies of spinal mechanics, White and Panjabi[5] have challenged the very usage of common clinical terms such as "flexion, compression, extension, torsion, bending, etc.," claiming that such motions simply can not and do not occur by themselves in the spine, but rather occur only as *coupled motions.* For example, lateral bending "involves rotations about the horizontal and vertical axes, respectively, as well as translation perpendicular to the sagittal plane. In other words, lateral bending may cause any combination of transverse shear in the horizontal plane, rotational shear about the vertical axis, and tensile and compressive stresses in the vertebral bodies. Therefore, to assume that a mechanism of injury involves only lateral bending is an oversimplification[5]."

All that now said and agreed with, what was true of our previous discussion of mechanisms of skull fracture (chapter 8) is true here too: 1) the most common things are most common, and 2) the probable kinematics of the occupant during an accident often defines what was possible, and therefore what most probably occurred.

If, for example, it was not probable that an occupant's spine was subjected to a compressive load in a given accident, then the presence of an anterior inferior vertebral body lip fracture is presumptive evidence of a hyperextension load as its cause. And if axial compression was possible but its presence was uncertain or undeterminable, then we must consider that *either* hyperflexion or hyperextension may have been the cause of an anterior inferior vertebral body lip fracture when it is seen on x-ray.

Fractures, Dislocations and Stability of the Musculoskeletal Spine

A major consideration in the treatment and outcome of *all* fractures and dislocations of the musculoskeletal spine is the concept of *stability* of the injured spine. As a general rule, stability from comparable injuries increases as we course from the head toward the foot, which is to say that a cervical injury is more liable to be unstable than is a lumbar injury. This is also to say that the types of crash injuries that occur in the neck are more likely of a nature that will be unstable than a crash injury of the low spine.

Determining the stability of the injured spine asks that the clinician determine (somehow) whether the damage to ligament and bone will result in such displacements under *future* physiologic loads that neurologic damage (or pain and/or deformity) will occur ("unstable") or will not occur ("stable").

This is very difficult to do. And the difficulty not withstanding, error in this determination may cause either unnecessary surgery or avoidable neurologic damage, loss of function(s), pain and deformity. Given these choices, I should be surprised if bias does not exist toward ready surgical intervention, since the alternative of neurologic loss, pain, etc. is so often a far greater risk and the determination of stability so often unclear. To me, at least, such bias is justifiable and remains under the umbrella of clinical judgement and experience, even though a variety of radiologic and clinical methods of evaluation of spinal stability exist for each of the spinal regions.

Injuries of The Upper Cervical Spine (C1, C2). In addition to the references for the spine already given above, all that you may want to know about the cervical spine is covered with remarkable thoroughness by a 1983 publication of *The Cervical Spine Research Society*[30].

The first cervical vertebra's engagement with the base of the skull is termed *the occipital-atlantal joint*. Injuries to this joint and the remaining cervical vertebrae most often occur because of a blow (or any load) to the head. (When head injuries are present trauma physicians will also examine and take x-rays of the neck.)

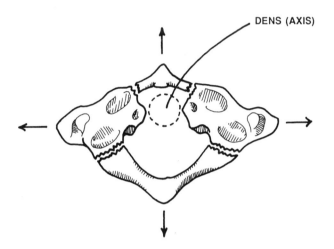

DENS (AXIS)

Figure 45
A COMMINUTED FRACTURE OF C1 (THE ''JEFFERSON FRACTURE'')

Pure compression originating at or applied to the vertex of the skull and transmitted along the long axis of the body (the y-axis) may cause the ring of C1 to burst into 4 fragments as the occipital condyles are driven into C1. The 4 fragments burst outward, away from the spinal cord.

The most typical appearance of such a fracture is shown above. It is termed a ''Jefferson Fracture'' after the man who described it and its mechanism of formation.

Fortunately, despite its location and its awful appearance, it is a relative benign injury, generally stable and only rarely involving any damage at all to the spinal cord.

Because the vertebral arteries pass through the lateral masses of C1, these arteries are at risk. Despite their vulnerable location, injuries to the vertebral arteries are reportedly quite rare in both Jefferson fractures and in similar fractures (from a similar mechanism) that involve only the posterior arch of C1.

Dislocation at this joint is reported as relatively rare and generally fatal. Presumably, it is due to anterior displacement of the skull relative to the atlas. However, both the mechanism and actual incidence of this injury is neither well studied or nor well known. Such injury appears to be often missed at autopsy, perhaps because pathologists rarely take radiographs of this area, being (apparently wrongly) confident of their ability to detect fractures and dislocations of C1 and C2 on palpation and inspection. In fact, in a few hundred fatal accidents that I have reviewed this past decade, I cannot recall a single example in which radiographs had been taken of an unhospitalized victim prior to autopsy as preparation for autopsy, and perhaps consequently, I can recall but 1 or 2 C1 and C1-C2 dislocations or fracture dislocations found at autopsy.

However, as indicated by a study of non-hospitalized traffic accident fatalities in which flexion/extension radiographs *were* taken prior to autopsy, *20 percent of all traffic accident fatalities had occipital-C1 or C1-C2 injuries*, with the occipital-atlantal joint injuries as the more common[31]. Which is to suggest that **in about one-of-every-five autopsies of traffic fatalities, occiput-C1 and C1-C2 dislocations and fractures are regularly and consistently being missed**. Try telling that to a forensic pathologist and note the look that you get in return.

Fractures of the first cervical vertebra most often involve either the posterior arch of C1 or are comminuted fractures of the entire ring of C1, the latter being termed a "Jefferson fracture," after G. Jefferson[32], figure 45. Both injuries appear to result from axial compression (from the head), the posterior arch fracture from compression directed somewhat posteriorly and the Jefferson fracture being vertical compression from the very vertex of the skull. Both of these fractures usually are surprisingly stable. Both fractures potentially involve the vertebral arteries with which they are in intimate contact, thus both injuries may cause symptoms of basilar artery insufficiency and may have vertebral artery complications of various sorts, from immediate death through aneurysm formation.

The *second cervical vertebra* also lacks a vertebral body, as does C1, but C2 has the prominent posterior vertical bony appendage, the *dens* (also termed the *odontoid*), which engages the posterior ring of the atlas thus allowing it to pivot about the dens and providing thereby the impressive degree of rotation about the long body axis which happens at the C1-C2 joint. (Note that almost no axial rotation can occur at the joint above, that of the occipital-atlantal joint.)

The dens fractures in any of three places: in the bony shaft of the dens, at the junction of the dens and the body of C2, and in the body of C2 itself. These are

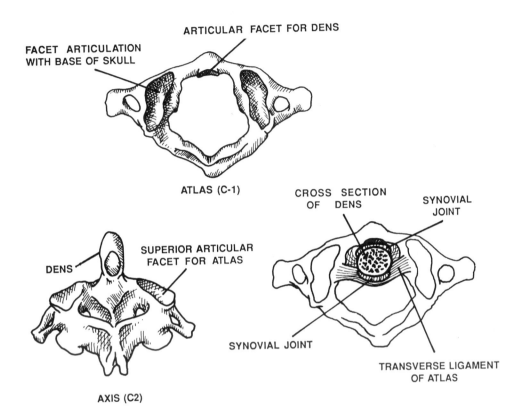

Figure 46
THE ATLANTO-AXIAL JOINT (C1-C2 JOINT)

The upper left figure is that of C1, as viewed from above (from the viewpoint of the base of the skull). The bone just below C1 is C2, viewed from the rear and slightly above.

The lower right hand illustration shows C1, again viewed from above, with C2 below it and the articulation of the dens (a tooth-like projection of C2) in its normal location within the anterior arch of C1.

Clearly, the C1-C2 joint is designed primarily for rotation to occur at that joint since it is the only spinal column articulation with a pivot post (the dens) as a primary articulation between two vertebrae. With the "post and ring" articulation of the dens it is somewhat surprising, to say the least, that *spontaneous dislocation* (i.e., dislocation apparently unrelated to trauma) is known to occur at this joint.

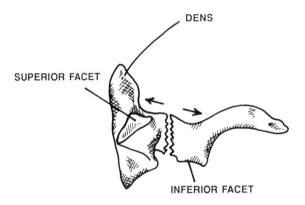

DENS

SUPERIOR FACET

INFERIOR FACET

C2 VERTEBRA (AXIS)

Figure 47
HANGMAN'S FRACTURE

This is an extension injury involving a fracture of the pars interarticularis (the bone between the facets) of C2; it is also called traumatic spondylolisthesis of C2.

When this fracture results from hanging it is due to tension and extension. When this fracture results from a diving accident or from car crash, it results from extension and compression at C2.

As with other injuries that have emotionally charged descriptor-names, such as "whiplash" sprain, the injury may be more simple than its name would suggest. For a hangman's fracture as a result of a diving impact or a car crash, not only doesn't the victim not die because of the injury, the victim usually doesn't have any neurologic symptoms of deficits. Treatment will vary with the extent of concurrent ligamentous damage which determines whether or not the fracture is stable. When stable, simple immobilization will often be all the treatment that is necessary.

termed Type I, II and III respectively, with Types I and III being relatively benign and Type II, fracture at the base of the dens, having a high rate of non-union and being considered therefore as a dangerous fracture. See figure 46 for the Atlanto-Axial joint.

Atlanto-Axial dislocations may be either *traumatic* or, somewhat remarkably to my mind, they may be *spontaneous* dislocations. Certainly it is not difficult to imagine trauma causing C1-C2 dislocations, but it is a fact that spontaneous dislocations at C1-C2, and dislocations from trivial trauma occur so often at this joint that a number of names have been applied to the atraumatic event, including such elegant terms as "malum subocciputale rheumaticum," and "torticollis nasopharyngien" as well as at least five other equally grotesque synonyms. Essentially spontaneous atlanto-axial dislocations result from inflammatory processes (as in the various forms of arthritis), regional bacterial and viral infections, as well as from the more obvious causes such as tumor growth and congenital growth anomalies (such as Down's syndrome). Treatment for the spontaneous dislocations is about the same as for traumatically induced dislocations,with potentially terrible consequences for the untreated cases and the missed diagnoses.

Hangman's fracture, which may also be termed *traumatic spondylolisthesis*, refers to a fracture occurring in the bone between any two articular facets of C2. (Figure 47.) In judicial hanging it happens because of a combination of extension and tension, while in diving accidents and in car crash, where it is not at all uncommon, extension and axial compression are its cause[33]. It is well described in a paper written about 80 years ago and charmingly entitled "The Ideal Lesion in Judicial Hanging," by Wood-Jones[34].

In the judicial setting the period of tension (hanging) is rather prolonged, assuring that there is plenty of time for dislocation to occur with its resultant (generally fatal) neurologic consequences. And, in the absence of the fatal neurologic consequences, the prolonged time epoch of the judicial setting assures that the alternative of simple strangulation will yield the desired end result should the neurologic trauma be insufficient for this purpose.

In vehicular trauma (and diving accidents) the time epoch is very brief and neurologic symptoms are often absent, perhaps because there is laxity of the neural arch with little or no displacement, or there is simply too little time for the loading to cause significant displacement[35].

I have dwelled on this fracture partly because it is intriguing (in a morbid sort of way) and partly because, when it is present in a car accident, attorneys and insurance adjusters seem so enthralled and overly impressed with the term "hangman's fracture" that they seem to run wild with what is simply another high cervical fracture, quite often stable and quite often without neurologic consequences in the car crash setting.

Injuries of The Lower Cervical Spine (C3-C7) occur to vertebrae more typically configured than the first two cervical vertebrae in that they have true vertebral bodies, which C1 and C2 do not have. Vertebral body fractures include compression fractures (both wedge and burst fractures) and the already-mentioned "tear drop fracture," (which in fact marks a fracture dislocation).

In the C3-7 region of the spine it is not uncommon to see only minimal residual displacement of the vertebral body in the presence of concurrent tetraplegia. Remember that the residual displacements seen in x-rays do not indicate the bony relationships that existed at the moment of peak load and peak displacement; radiographs show only where things ended up *after* the injury occurred.

Facet dislocations occur relatively easily in the lower cervical region because the facet joints are at about 45 degrees to the plane of the vertebrae. The progressively greater vertical angle of the facets below the cervical spine makes for progressively less probable facet dislocation in the lower spine.

Facet dislocations may be either unilateral or bilateral, may be either "perched" or "locked," and may be associated with other vertebral fractures, including facet fractures. Unilateral facet dislocations occur when lateral bending is forced: the coupled axial rotation that normally occurs with lateral bending tears posterior ligaments as the spinous process rotates toward the convexity of the bend and the facet on the same (convex) side goes too far forward and dislocates. If the superior facet is trapped forward but still on top of the inferior facet, it is termed "perched;" if it is dropped forward of the inferior facet it is effectively locked in that position and is termed a "locked facet." Bilateral facet dislocations may occur when a severe tensile load on the posterior elements is coupled with a forward or flexing motion of the superior vertebra. They too may perch, but more commonly they lock. Clearly, for such dislocation to occur there has had to be considerable tearing of intervertebral ligaments and joint instability is a common consequence of dislocated facets. See figure 48 for the appearance of a pair of locked facets.

Below C2, vehicular trauma and its attendant high forces make for a variety of dislocations and fracture dislocations. These injuries commonly are neurologic

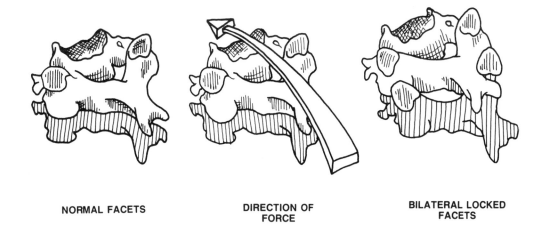

NORMAL FACETS   **DIRECTION OF FORCE**   **BILATERAL LOCKED FACETS**

Figure 48
BILATERAL PERCHED AND LOCKED FACETS

As shown here the facets of the upper vertebra not only dislocated forward to be on top of the facets of the lower vertebra (*"perched"*), they continued to slide forward until they dropped in front of and *locked* against the facets of the vertebra below them. When they were perched on top of the lower vertebra's superior facets they were termed "perched" facets. This injury of course cannot occur unless there has been extensive disruption of the intervertebral ligaments, which lead us to expect that this dislocation is unstable.

As the arrow above indicates, this dislocation results from a considerable force exerted and directed both upward and forward.

Unilateral facet dislocations also are most common in the lower cervical vertebrae, where the facets form about a 45 degree angle to the horizontal.

catastrophies, causing great spinal cord damage, although there are the usual exceptions that make us wonder how and even why they were excepted.

The cervical injuries noted above have flexion as a primary causal component of fracture and/or fracture dislocation. When extension is a primary force then sprains are more usual than fracture or subluxation.

In our society cervical extension sprains occur most often when the unrestrained head of a car occupant is inertially (and relatively) displaced rearward, as when his car is struck from the rear by another vehicle. This event is inaccurately albeit colorfully described as a "whiplash injury" which it certainly is not.

What it *is* should be termed a "cervical sprain," a term less colorful but more descriptive of the usual event. Acceleration induced hyperextension on occasion also causes more severe injuries, such as subluxations of the vertebral bodies and of the posterior joints[36]. Additional other hyperextension induced pathology has often been suggested to explain what occasionally appears to be bizarre complaints, such as tinnitus, dysphagia, and blurring of vision, all or any of which may continue months or years after the injury was incurred.

Two different studies done a decade apart and philosophically even further apart shared the same results, that *about 12 percent of severe cervical acceleration induced extension injuries (cervical sprains) had "significant" disability even after the passage of several years, even after any possible litigation related gain no longer existed*[37] [38].

Crash injuries involving the thoracic vertebrae are often violent events in which the flexed spinal column is additionally subjected to coupled forces of rotation and/or lateral bending. It is usual to find spinal cord damage, with concurrent severely torn posterior ligaments, fractured: facets, pars interarticularis, laminae, transverse processes and the like. Nearly half of all of the spinal cord injuries from motor vehicle crash will occur in the thoracic spine[3].

It would seem that the splint-like bracing provided by the ribs should reduce the displacements of thoracic vertebrae, but the high incidence of spinal cord injuries noted above suggests that any splinting effects of the rib cage do not function to prevent either injuries or subluxations, but rather serve to attenuate the post-accident appearance of the injuries which so often is more benign than the spinal injury sustained. While these injuries are usually unstable, they usually are not as grossly displaced in their appearance as are, say, comparable cervical injuries.

Ejections from particularly violent collisions and from the more common rollovers may cause wedge fractures or burst fractures of the vertebral bodies, similar to those more often found in accidental falls. (In NHTSA's 1990 Fatal Accident Reporting

System about 14 percent of occupants involved in fatal crashes were ejected, representing double that percentage of the total of occupant fatalities.)

The typical *wedge fracture* of the thoraco-lumbar spine is less than about 30 percent of the height of the vertebral body. If it *is* less than say, a 30 percent compression, it usually is a benign, stable fracture of little consequence either acutely or as a disability. That this fracture is of little consequence is clear from the *1988 AMA Guide to the Evaluation of Permanent Impairment* which allows only 2 percent impairment of the whole person for a 25 percent compression of a thoracic vertebral body.

Burst fractures are compression fractures from more axially aligned loading than is true of wedge fractures. The endplate collapses and the intervertebral disc is driven into the vertebral body, literally bursting it apart and driving fragments of cancellous bone in all directions. When the anterior and posterior longitudinal ligaments remain intact the injury is stable; when one or more of these ligaments is torn it not only is an unstable injury, but bony fragments may pass through and harm major blood vessels anterior to the fracture or, more commonly, bony fragments are driven rearward, into the spinal canal and/or the spinal cord itself. In the thoracic spine, the spinal cord may be injured; in the lumbar spine, the cauda equina may be injured.

In my experience somewhere around one-half of all thoracic wedge fractures and fracture dislocations, from about T4 on down, occurred when the flexed thorax was struck or loaded from either the lower cervical or upper thoracic regions.

Lateral wedge fractures result from lateral bending with axial compression. They are unlike flexion compression fractures in that they more frequently result in impairment. They are often associated with concurrent fractures of a facet, or of a pedicle, or of a transverse process, any or all occurring on the same side as the apex of the wedge.

Lower thoracic and lumbar fractures and fracture dislocations will be dealt with together because their crash injuries are somewhat similar and because crash injuries of the musculoskeletal spine concentrate at the thoracolumbar junction[3].

The thoracic spine is stiffer than the lumbar spine[39], and an additional somewhat abrupt change occurs as well in the orientation of the articular facets of the lumbar spine as compared to the orientation of the thoracic facets; we have earlier noted that facets' orientations largely govern what motions are possible in a given segment.

The last two thoracic vertebrae are transitional. They have "floating ribs," which is to say that the lower two ribs are attached posteriorly to the last two vertebrae but are not attached to anything anteriorly. The last thoracic vertebra (T12) is usually an even more transitional vertebra than T11 in that it has but two costal facets for the twelfth rib rather than 4, and while T12's superior articular processes (superior facets) resemble thoracic facets in facing essentially posteriorly, its inferior facets resemble those of the lumbar region, facing laterally and anteriorly. (The preceding discussion on the transitional nature of T11, T12 should be taken with a grain of statistical salt. Biological variation being what it is, transition from thoracic to lumbar facet orientation in fact may occur anywhere from T9 to L1.)

Compression fractures, as were discussed above, are most frequent in the lower thoracic and upper lumbar vertebral bodies and the majority are wedge fractures. They may be caused either by an eccentrically (anteriorly) located compressive force or by a combination of flexion (bending forward) and of compression, the latter combination being by far the more common in car crashes in my experience. They do not seem to cause significant problems or impairment until the compression exceeds 30 to 50 percent of the vertebrae.

Fractures and fracture dislocations in the thoracolumbar region require very large forces to happen at all, since the lower thoracic and the lumbar vertebrae are quite large, strong bones with large, strong ligaments that are not easily torn or broken. Occasionally, fractures and fracture dislocations occur in this region and involve only the posterior elements, as *fractures of the neural arch*. These fractures are easy to miss unless they are actively looked for in good quality radiographs. Because they are frequently associated with transverse process fractures, they should be looked for when the more easily seen transverse process is present. Neural arch fractures may result from axial loading combined with hyperextension and/or from axial torsion with flexion[40]. Incidentally, fractures of the thoracolumbar transverse processes have a rather high association with trauma of abdominal viscera, (about 20 percent), with associated pelvic fractures (29 percent) and with additional spinal fractures, (about 15 percent)[41].

Lap belt induced fractures and fracture dislocations are a special case. This could be discussed in the chapter concerned with restraint systems, but we'll deal with such injuries here because of the remarkable variation in injuries that result from essentially the same loading, that of hyperflexion of the thoracolumbar spine over and around the abdominally located seat belt.

Let me first emphasize that the lap belt should *never* be located anywhere but over

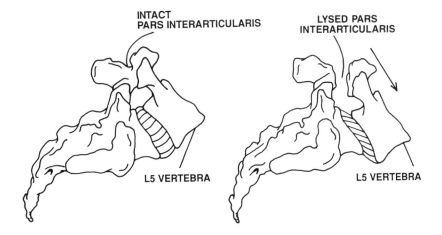

INTACT
PARS INTERARTICULARIS

LYSED PARS
INTERARTICULARIS

L5 VERTEBRA

L5 VERTEBRA

Figure 49
SPONDYLOLYSIS AND SPONDYLOLISTHESIS

This curious separation of bone occurring at the pars interarticularis (see diagrams above) has a probable genetic origin and a possible traumatic origin as well.

The probable genetic origin is suggested by a very high incidence of occurrence in certain racial groups and the possible traumatic origin is suggested by the higher than usual incidence in certain sports activities, such as gymnastics.

Once the pars is lysed or fractured (i.e., spondylolysis), the forward-tilted lumbar vertebral body will, as it were, slide forward (i.e., spondylolisthesis).

Spondylolysis and subsequent spondylolisthesis, you will certainly want to know, also has been found to have an unusually high occurrence rate in Dachshunds as compared to other breeds. I mention this because it also would seem to support the genetic argument as the basis for most spondylolysis and spondylolisthesis.

the bony pelvis, at the anterior superior spines of the ilia of the pelvis, to be exact. In what well may be the most unambiguous and clear statement ever made by the National Highway Traffic Safety Administration in any of their so-called safety standards, they said [49 CFR Ch. V, section 571-209, S4.1(b)], "A seat belt assembly shall provide pelvis restraint whether or not upper torso restraint is provided, and *the pelvic restraint shall be designed to remain on the pelvis under all conditions including collision or roll-over of the motor vehicle.*" (I have added the italics.) But because of many factors, especially that of maldesign of the lap belt attachment locations[42], seat belts slide up over occupants' pelvic anterior superior prominences, and/or occupants slide under seat belts, allowing them to hyperflex around the lap belt webbing, causing tensile loading to the vertebral column at, above and below the webbing[43]. This 1969 paper notes that *this same load* may cause disruption of the posterior elements that may be "osseous, ligamentous, or both" and that there may be little or no wedging, forward or lateral displacement of the superior fragment or vertebra. In addition, the disruption most often was between L1 to L3 and seat belt contusions were often visible on the abdomen.

What a variety of responses to a singular load.

White and Panjabi[5] were so struck by this variation in response to hyperflexion by the thoracolumbar spine that they were tempted "to present a *law* of mechanism of injury. ***Similar force patterns do not necessarily produce identical failure patterns.***" While there may have been some tongue-in-cheek, (at least I believe so), they were emphasizing that whether ligament or bone fails first under a given load will depend upon 1) individual variation in strength of materials and 2) the time epoch of the loading, since both bone and ligament are viscoelastic materials (as we have previously noted in chapter 3) and their failure in tensile load is necessarily time-dependent.

Spondylolysis and spondylolisthesis are terms not to be confused with *spondolysis*, the latter term referring to the bony spurs that form on vertebral body junctions with intervertebral discs in degenerative joint disease of the vertebrae, as discussed above.

Spondylolysis refers to a fracture or otherwise-caused loss of the vertebral isthmus (also called the pars interarticularis, the bone segment that separates the facets). See figure 49 for spondylolysis and spondylolisthesis.

Spondylolisthesis refers to the slipping forward of one vertebral body on another, which usually occurs at the weakest link in the vertebral column, the lumbosacral joint (i.e., L5-S1) as a result of spondylolysis. It is a strange looking lesion wherein L5 literally slides down the inclined and forward tilting surface of S1. The amount of sliding is of course limited by the several ligaments that bind these vertebrae together as well as by the paravertebral muscles that also surround this joint. The paravertebral muscle spasm and the stretch of intervertebral muscles are believed to be the source of pain that this condition engenders[7].

All in all, spondylolysis and its subsequent spondylolisthesis are conditions whose origins are less than clear. A genetic element may be supposed from the 2 percent or so incidence in American Blacks, the near 6 percent incidence in American Whites and the 60 percent incidence (!) in American Eskimos[5]. Although most spondylolysis appears to occur from genetic and other factors, such as "fatigue fractures," (primarily in athletes whose specialties are uniquely repetitive, such as gymnasts), singular traumatic events are known to cause these lesions[44].

In order to claim an acute traumatic source for spondylolysis it should be shown that there was: 1) antecedent severe trauma, 2) the irregular edges of a "new" fracture seen on initial radiographs, and 3) abundant callus formation on subsequent radiographs[44]. Only 10 cases or so of acute traumatic spondylolysis have been reported in the open literature.

Sacral and coccygeal fractures also are high force fractures. The sacral fractures may be classified as 1) in conjunction with a pelvic fracture (and most generally vertically aligned), 2) an isolated fracture of the lower sacral segments (generally a transverse fracture) and 3) an isolated fracture of the upper sacral segments (and also generally transversely aligned)[45]. **"The frequency of each type of fracture decreases from (1) to (3), but the neurologic implications increase.**[45]" The second type appears to be from a direct blow to the sacrum: the third type from an indirect blow. The first type may be attributable to whatever mechanism fractured the pelvis.

Coccygeal fractures are neurologically trivial injuries with essentially no implications of permanent impairment, so we will say little else about them.

Injuries of the Spinal Cord

General

About 2,500 BC a papyrus was written that some 4,500 years later came to be known as the "Edwin Smith Surgical Papyrus[46]." In so many words, it said that spinal injury is a class of injury not worth treating because no treatment alters the outcome.

There still is reason to believe that this may be so. With the exceptions of treating

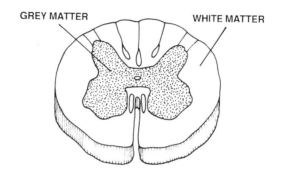

FRONT (ANTERIOR)

GREY MATTER   WHITE MATTER

BACK (POSTERIOR)

Figure 50
A SLICE OF THE SPINAL CORD

This is a diagrammatic, simplified drawing of a transverse slice through the spinal cord about at the level of the lumbar enlargement, much as if one took a slice of a sausage and looked down at it.

There is a central gray area described by anatomists of pleasant associations as resembling a butterfly in shape. It is largely composed of neuroglia, which is a connective nervous tissue and of neurons, which are the nerve cells themselves.

The surrounding white matter consists largely of transverse sections of communicating nerve fibers, the axons of nerves, and their individual surrounding sheaths of a fatty substance termed myelin. The axonal nerve fibers are analogous to communicating wires; their myelin sheaths are analogous to insulation around the wires.

(These analogies are crude ones and should not be literally construed, for nerve fibers are not wires and, unlike wires, nerve transmissions are biochemical events as well as electrical events.)

concomitant respiratory or circulatory failure (which we would have to do anyway), and perhaps also of decompressing the spinal cord by realigning grossly misaligned and/or unstable dislocations and fracture dislocations, little that we do today is known to influence the recovery or lack of recovery of nervous system tissue once it has been traumatized. We cannot, for example, sew the spinal cord back together where it is torn apart and expect the torn nerves to once again transmit their "messages" as, for example, we can resplice a torn telephone cable and fully restore its function, fiber by fiber.

At this time about a quarter of a million of our citizens are permanently paralyzed from spinal cord trauma.

That this is still so is not to say that the pathophysiology of spinal cord trauma has not been the subject of intense and continuing world-wide investigation. Rather, that this is so despite so much study is testimony only to the complexity and difficulty of the subject.

While spinal cord injuries do have surgical and pharmacologic treatments, the efficacy of early surgical intervention (especially the first four hours) and a variety of vaso-affective and metabolic drugs has yet to be established. A variety of treatments have come and gone, waxing because of some appealing theoretic basis, then waning as the clinical setting and the test of time have not provided support for the treatment. But as of today, as I sit here at my word processor, nothing known to our inventory of treatments seems to alter the progression of changes of structure and function that so inexorably follows trauma to the spinal cord.

To the general references listed under the above heading of Spinal Trauma, let me add *Spinal Injury*[47] by David Yashon and *Spinal Cord Monitoring*[48], edited by Schramm and Jones, and *The Pathophysiology of Spinal Trauma*[49], edited by R. Wilkins. These books have good overviews of the pathophysiology of spinal cord trauma and repair. I have used them as well as other references previously given for much of the following abbreviated presentation of this complex subject.

Anatomy of the Spinal Cord

As you will recall, the spinal cord occupies the spinal canal from the level of the C1 to L1-L2. There are two fusiform, thickened regions: the cervical enlargement (from C3 to T2) which accepts the additional neurons necessary for supplying the cervical and brachial plexuses, and the lumbosacral enlargement (from T9-10 to L1-2), for the additional neurons supplying the lumbosacral (i.e., lower limb) plexus.

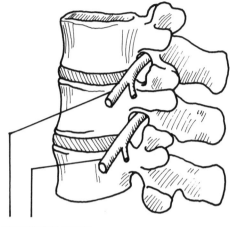

NERVE ROOTS EMERGING FROM
LUMBAR INVERTEBRAL FORAMINA

Figure 51
NERVE ROOTS EMERGING FROM INTERVERTEBRAL FORAMINA

Nerve rootlets emerge from the spinal cord on the ventral (front) and dorsal (back) portions of the cord, briefly merging into a single trunk as they pass through the foramina (Latin for "holes"), as shown above.

The size of the holes (intervertebral foramina) is easily and often reduced ("stenosed") with resultant compromise of the emerging nerve. Let us first look at what the holes are made of.

in front (anteriorly), by the body of the vertebra and the intervertebral disc;

above (superiorly), by the lower surface of the pedicle of the neural arch;

behind (posteriorly or dorsally) by the facet joint, and finally,

below (inferiorly), by the upper surface of the pedicle of the vertebra below.

Even a short list of sources of constriction of intervertebral foramina must include: 1) extreme bulging (if the foramen is already stenosed) or herniation of an intervertebral disc, 2) bony outgrowths from the posterior margins of the vertebral bodies (exostoses or bony spurs), and 3) osteoarthritic distortions of the pedicles or the facet joints.

In fact, many of these sources of foraminal constriction are related and typically will occur together, as in oseoarthritis causing synovial joint (facet) overgrowth and excessive motion at the facet joint, which in turn causes the formation of bony spurs and exostoses at the disc margins as the intervertebral joint is now too frequently hyperextended, which in turn causes disc disease and possible subsequent herniation of the disc's nucleus pulposus, etc.

Of course, it is the constriction of the foraminal opening that "pinches," if you will, the emerging spinal nerve and causes both motor and sensory problems at the nerve's terminations.

A transverse section through the spinal cord at almost any level will show a laterally bilobate, essentially round appearance, with a somewhat grayish "H" or butterfly shaped central area and a whitish region that largely surrounds the butterfly; see figure 50. Of course, the gray region is "gray matter," which we know to be neurons, and the whitish region is largely composed of myelinated ascending and descending nerve fibers, preponderantly organized into tracts or bundles. These tracts or vertical columns of nerve fibers (white matter) are precisely localizable within any spinal level and provide the basis for defining the location of lesions within the spinal cord by the tracts of fibers involved and a working knowledge of their function(s).

There are 31 pairs of spinal nerve roots that emerge from the lateral aspect of the spine. The posterior (dorsal) roots are sensory in function while the anterior (ventral) roots are motor in function. They merge to become a resultant pair of mixed nerves (i.e., sensory and motor functions in each nerve bundle), emerging through the intervertebral foramina, as seen in figure 51, servicing muscle, skin, and similar terminal organs and tissues at each level.

The spinal cord enjoys a rich and complex blood supply, but let us think of the blood supply in terms of the arterial supply, the microcirculation (arterioles, capillary beds and venules) and the venous drainage of the spinal cord, because trauma preponderantly involving each of these circulations seems to cause quite different patterns of cord injuries[48].

Spinal Cord Trauma

As with all other soft tissues, spinal cord trauma may involve any combination of compression, contusion and laceration from both direct injury to neurons and their axons as well as direct injury to their local blood vessels.

In the central nervous system the direct injuries just listed above are followed by a complex chain of initial events, termed *ischemia* (inadequate regional blood flow), subsequent *edema* (capillary leakage and local swelling) and later hemorrhagic necrosis of the cord (death of the cells and their axons, surrounded by leaked blood).

Of course, it is not that simple. There are numerous and various local tissue factors, such as regional catecholamines (adrenaline-like compounds) as well as other classes of tissue-released cytotoxins that appear to be impugned in adversely altering blood flow and tissue survival in injured central nervous tissue. Which is to say that local tissue-related chemicals are an important part of the ischemia/edema/hemorrhagic necrosis pattern involved in the death of spinal cord nervous tissue.

The pharmacologic treatments of cord trauma are attempts to inhibit a cascade of apparently inappropriate vascular responses produced within the cord by trauma to the spinal cord. Some of the drugs act directly on the blood vessels themselves; other drugs attempt to alter the production of edema or inhibit the destruction of the myelin nerve sheaths and so forth. For example, reserpine, a drug with considerable anti-adrenergic activity, appears to protect against traumatic hemorrhagic necrosis of the cord[49]. It is but one of a number of agents which appear to have both a rational basis for use in spinal cord injury and a low or negligible capacity to do harm. Although usage of such drugs, especially the use of corticosteroids and either mannitol or urea, are not really experimental, proof of their efficacy is not yet sufficient. Further, in light of the usually impaired circulation at the spinal cord injury site, there is good reason to believe that these drugs are delivered almost everywhere within the body except to those areas of the injured spinal cord where they are most needed.

Permanent paraplegia is due to permanent damage to the white matter, the myelinated axons in various spinal tracts. The time course of the impairment of blood flow to white matter clearly is paramount to the final outcome of white matter, i.e., whether or not white matter survives. About an hour after spinal cord trauma the blood flow to white matter is impaired. If it returns to normal within about a day, the paraplegia generally will be only transient; if the blood flow continues to decrease after 24 hours, the paraplegia will probably be permanent[50].

It has been our inability to alter the time course of destruction of the white matter that has been the basis of our inability to alter the outcome of spinal cord trauma.

Finally, as if our inability to alter the outcome of spinal cord trauma was not enough cause for frustration, there are a variety of adverse post traumatic myelopathies, continuing and progressive changes that may not be manifest for years after the trauma was incurred. Examples include *arachnoiditis*, a chronic progressive disorder, often causing such problems as spastic paralysis years after an injury that caused bleeding into the arachnoid space, and *syringomyelia*, another progressive paralytic complication due to cavity formation within the cord, following by months to years an episode of hemorrhagic necrosis within the cord. It is irreversible and only partly treatable by surgery.

The bleak picture of spinal cord injury is verified by the statistics of such injuries that have caused paralysis. For *complete quadriplegia* the death rate was 12 times normal, for *complete paraplegia* nearly 5 times normal and for partial "plegias" from 1 to 3 times normal[51]. This is for a calculated prevalence of at least 100,000 patients now alive in the U.S. with traumatic spinal cord injury, of whom about 40,000 have complete paralysis: 35,000 with complete lower limb paralysis and about 5,000 with complete paralysis of all four limbs. Some estimates have over 250,000 spinal cord injury victims living in the U.S. with about 10,000 new injuries added each year[47].

SUMMARY

We have considered both the importance and the vulnerability of the spine in terms of the frequency of its being a problem and the types of problems it may cause.

The anatomy of the spine was then considered from the viewpoint of its three functions, that of providing axial skeletal support, that of providing protection to the important and easily damaged spinal cord, and that of its remarkable flexibility, allowing a considerable range of skeletal motions. The intervertebral disk and its age related expected degenerative changes were discussed in some detail because of the discs' medical, surgical and litigation related popularity.

Spinal trauma was dealt with in terms of musculoskeletal trauma patterns as well as the mechanical stability of spinal musculoskeletal injuries, and later and briefly, in terms of injury to the spinal cord proper.

We were distressed by our inability to do very much, at this time as in the past, to change the course of healing of spinal cord injuries when once they have been incurred.

BIBLIOGRAPHY

1. Wiesel, S.W., Feffer, H.L., Borenstein, D.G. and R.H. Rothman: *Industrial Low Back Pain.* 2nd ed. Michie, Charlottesville, 1989.
2. Cailliet, R.: *Low Back Pain Syndrome.* 4th ed. Davis, Philadelphia, 1989.
3. Fife, D. and J. Kraus: Anatomic location of spinal cord injury. *Spine 11*:2, 1986.
4. Anderson, D.W. and R.L. McLaurin, Eds.: Report on the national head and spinal cord injury survey. *J Neurosurg, 53*:1, 1980.
5. White, A.A. and M.M. Panjabi: *Clinical Biomechanics of the Spine.* Lippincott, Philadelphia, 1978.
6. Nachemson, A.: Lumbar interdiscal pressure. *Acta Orthop Scand Suppl 43*, 1960.
7. Kapandji, I.A.: *The Physiology of the Joints.* vol III, Churchill Livingstone, New York, 1974.
8. Gardner, E., Gray, D.J. and R. O'Rahilly: *Anatomy.* Saunders, Philadelphia, 1975.
9. Virgin, W.: Experimental investigations into physical properties of intervertebral disc. *J Bone Joint Surg [Br], 33B*:607, 1951.
10. Hirsch, C.: The reaction of intervertebral discs to compression forces. *J Bone Joint Surg 37A [Am]*:1188, 1955.
11. Adams, M.A. and W.C. Hutton: Prolapsed intervertebral disc. A hyperflexion injury. *Spine 7*:184, 1982.
12. Adams, M.A. and W.C. Hutton: Gradual disc prolapse. *Spine 10*:524, 1985.
13. Kelsey, J.L., Githens, P.B., White II, A.A., Holford, T.R., Walters, S.D., O'Connor, T., Ostfeld, A.M., Weil, U., Southwick, W.O. and J.A. Calogero: An epidemiologic study of lifting and twisting on the job and risk for acute prolapsed lumbar intervertebral disc. *J Orthop Res 2*:61, 1984.
14. Goel, V.K., Voo, L.M., Weinstein, J.N., Kiu, Y.K., Okuma, T. and G.O. Njus: Response of the ligamentous lumbar spine to cyclic bending loads. *Spine 13*:294, 1988.
15. Farfan, J.F., Cossette, J.W., Robertson, H.G., Wells, R.V. and H. Kraus: The effects of torsion on the lumbar intervertebral joints; the role of torsion in the production of disc degeneration. *J Bone Joint Surg [Am], 52A*:468, 1970.
16. Perry, O.: Fracture of the vertebral end-plate in the lumbar spine. *Acta Orthop Scan Suppl 25*, 1957.

17. Roaf, R.: A study of the mechanics of spinal injuries. *J Bone Joint Surg [Br] 42B*:810, 1960.

18. Rolander, S.D. and W.E. Blair: Deformation and fracture of the lumbar vertebral end-plate. *Orthop Clin North Am 6*:75, 1975.

19. Koeller, W., Muehlhaus, W., Meier, W. and F. Hartmann: Biomechanical properties of human intervertebral discs subjected to axial dynamic compression — influence of age and degeneration. *J Biomech 19*:807, 1986.

20. Hittelsberger, W.E. and R.M. Witten: Abnormal myelograms in asymptomatic patients. *J Neurosurg 28*:204, 1968.

21. Weisel, S.W., Tsourmas, N., Feffer, H.L., Citrin, C.M. and N. Patronas: A study of computer-assisted tomography I. The incidence of positive CAT scans in an asymptomatic group of patients. *Spine 9*:549, 1984.

22. Salter, R.B.: *Textbook of Disorders and Injuries of the Musculoskeletal System.* 2nd ed. Williams & Wilkins, Baltimore, 1983.

23. Armstrong, J.R.: *Lumbar Disc Lesions.* Williams & Wilkins, Baltimore, 1965.

24. Weber, H.: Lumbar disc herniations. A prospective study of prognostic factors including a controlled trial. *J Oslo City Hosp 28*:33, 89, 1978.

25. Spangfort, E.V.: The lumbar disc herniation. A computer-aided analysis of 2,504 operations. *Acta Orthop Scand Suppl 142*:61, 1972.

26. Mcnab, I.: *Backache.* Williams & Wilkins, Baltimore, 1977.

27. Rothman, R.R. and F.A. Simeone: *The Spine.* 2nd ed. Saunders, Philadelphia, 1982.

28. Ghista, D.N. and H. Frankel: *Spinal Cord Injury Medical Engineering.* Thomas, Springfield, 1986.

29. Gosch, H.H., Gooding, E. and R.C. Schneider: An experimental study of cervical spine and cord injuries. *J Trauma 12*:570, 1972.

30. The Cervical Spine Research Society: *The Cervical Spine.* Lippincott, Philadelphia, 1983.

31. Alker Jr., G.J., Oh, Y.S., Leslie, E.V., Lehotay, J., Panaro, V.A. and E.G. Eschner: Post mortem radiology of head and neck injuries in fatal traffic accidents. *J Neuroadiol 114*:611, 1975.

32. Jefferson, G.: Fracture of the atlas vertebra, report of four cases and a review of those previously recorded. *Br J Surg 7*:407, 1920.

33. Williams, T.G.: Hangman's fracture. *J Bone Joint Surg [Br] 57B*:82, 1975.

34. Wood-Jones, F.: The ideal lesion produced by judicial hanging. *Lancet I*:53, 1913.

35. Payne, E.E. and J.D. Spillane: The cervical spine. *Brain 80*:571, 1957.
36. Jackson, R.: *The Cervical Syndrome.* 2nd ed. Thomas, Springfield, 1958.
37. Gotten, N.: Survey of one hundred cases of whiplash injury after settlement of litigation. *JAMA 162*:856, 1956.
38. Macnab, I.: Acceleration injuries of the cervical spine. *J Bone Joint Surg [Am] 46A*:1979, 1964.
39. Panjabi, M.M., Brand, R.M. and A.A. White: Three-dimensional flexibility and stiffness properties of the human thoracic spine. *J Biomech 9*:185, 1976.
40. Sullivan, J.D. and J.F. Farfan: The crumpled neural arch. *Orthop Clin N Am 6*:199, 1975.
41. Sturm, J.T. and J.F. Perry: Injuries associated with fractures of the transverse processes of the thoracic and lumbar vertebrae. *J Trauma 24*:597, 1984.
42. Leung, Y.C., Tarriere, C., Lestrelin, D., Got, C., Guillon, F., Patel, A. and J. Hureau: Submarining injuries of 3-pt. belted occupants in frontal collisions — description, mechanisms and protection. *SAE* paper 821158, 1982.
43. Smith, W.S. and H. Kaufer: Patterns and mechanisms of lumbar injuries associated with lap seat belts. *J Bone Joint Surg [Am] 51A*:2, 1969.
44. Cope, R.: Acute traumatic spondylolysis. *Clin Orthop 230*:162, 1988.
45. Sabiston, C.P. and P.C. Wing: Sacral fractures: classification and neurologic implications. *J Trauma 26*:1113, 1986.
46. Breasted, J.H.: *The Edwin Smith Surgical Papyrus,* vol. 1, U Chicago Press, Chicago, 1957.
47. Yashon, D.: *Spinal Injury.* 2nd ed., Appleton, Norwalk, 1986.
48. Schramm, J. and S.J. Jones (Ed.): *Spinal Cord Monitoring.* Springer-Verlag, Berlin, 1985.
49. Osterholm, J.L.: *The Pathophysiology of Spinal Trauma.* R. Wilkins, ed., Thomas, Springfield, 1978.
50. Dohrman, G.J., Wagner, F.C. and P.C. Bucy: The microvasculature in transitory traumatic paraplegia: an electron microscopic study in the monkey. *J Neurosurg 35*:263, 1971.
51. Breithaupt, D.J., Jousse, A.T. and M. Wynne-Jones: Late causes of death and life expectancy in paraplegia. *Can Med Assoc J 85*:73, 1961.

CHAPTER 10

___

SEAT BELTS AND OTHER RESTRAINTS: WHAT THEY CAN DO; WHAT THEY CANNOT DO; HOW THEY CAN HELP AND HOW THEY CAN HURT

THE PROBLEM IS . . .

There is a limited space through which a restrained occupant may flail without striking some portion of the interior of the car. This space is termed the "flail space" in chapter 2 and it is illustrated in figures 4, 5, and 6 of that chapter.

We would like to enlarge the flail volume allowed each occupant so that contact or the probability of contact with the vehicle interior during crash is lessened. However, the option to enlarge the flail space is a limited option in that we can only enlarge it so much before the resultant flail volume becomes so large that it would likely be larger than a typical car's entire interior volume.

The problem then is to design some system of webbing or of other devices which either

- limits occupant motion and displacement so that there is no contact with the car's interior, or
- restrains major body segments, so that contact with interior surfaces is limited only to the mass of whatever body segment contacts an interior surface rather than the mass of the entire free-flying body (which is pretty much what we try to do now), or
- substantially reduces interior contact force, as by padding all interior probable crash contact surfaces with energy absorbing material so that the force loading of occupant-to-interior contact is lowered enough to prevent serious injuries.

An air bag, for example, is both a device to reduce displacement and an energy absorbing contact surface, all in one.

In this chapter we will look to restraints and other systems intended to reduce injury. In the next chapter we will look at how we measure or define what a "serious injury" is, since what is serious with respect to threat-to-life is not necessarily even related to what is serious with respect to subsequent impairment and disability.

GENERAL

Restraint systems do just and only just what their name says they do: they restrain. They restrain motion. They do not prevent motion or displacement; they restrain them. And the restraint applies primarily to those directions that it was specifically designed to restrain motion and displacement.

For the lap belt portion of the most usual webbing restraint (the three-point or lap/chest belt), motion or displacement is restrained for all directions except downward and rearward. For the diagonal chest restraint, motion or displacement is restrained only forward, upward and outward (the direction from which the belts retract).

Thus for the most common frontal impact, the left-front-to-left-front impact, the right front occupant is thrown leftward and forward, and may be thrown out of the shoulder harness webbing since the webbing only crosses the right shoulder and not the left shoulder. For a right frontal impact the opposite is true; the driver is thrown rightward and forward, and again likely out of the shoulder harness webbing, thus again reducing the restraint to a lapbelt equivalent.

Since NHTSA's New Car Assessment Program (NCAP) tests are pure frontal barrier collisions we would not expect to see the loss of the diagonal chest harness which commonly occurs in right and left frontal oblique and lateral collisions. Let us then be appropriately surprised that in the first 150 NCAP frontal barrier crash tests rotation about the body's long axis (Z axis) was common, causing at least 4 of the dummies not only to twist completely out of their chest harnesses, but to strike the instrument panel (dash) with their heads as well. A second shoulder restraint (a "four point" system) would prevent the loss of torso restraint in angled frontal crashes.

How much do restraint systems restrain motion? For the average male driver in a 30 mile per hour frontal barrier collision the common three-point restrained chest will move forward about 10 to 13 inches despite the presence of the chest harness. The head will move forward some 19 to 24 inches, in a forward and downward arc[1][2][3]. Arms and lower legs (and the head) all are unrestrained and therefore they can and do flail about, driven by inertial forces that are unopposed, even as the surfaces they may contact are essentially unpadded. Knees move forward from 4 inches up

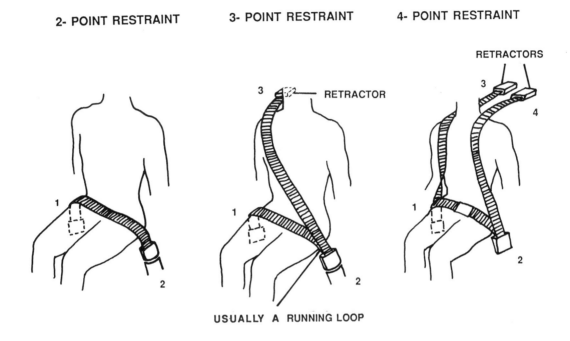

2- POINT RESTRAINT   3- POINT RESTRAINT   4- POINT RESTRAINT

USUALLY A RUNNING LOOP

Figure 52
TWO, THREE AND FOUR POINT RESTRAINT SYSTEMS

The number of "points" in the title description of webbing restraint systems refers, of course, to the number of *attachment points* used in a particular webbing restraint system, as should be clear from this illustration.

Five and 6 point restraints usually add attachment points for webbing located between the legs and designed to hold the lap belt portion of the restraint from riding up over the anterior superior iliac spines of the pelvis. Between-the-legs webbing attached to the lap belt also should prevent "submarining," which we have previously described as sliding forward, under the lap belt.

There are many, many other published designs for webbing restraints not shown here. Some use "Y" shaped webbings, others have woven net restraint vests gathered into webbings, and so forth. While the large number of other clever restraint mechanisms have not been shown here, I believe that the reader has gotten the message: we are far from exhausting all of what may be possible in the field of restraint system design, and that what we have now may not be the best of what we could have in the way of convenient and effective restraint systems.

to about 9 inches, because the pelvis slides forward that amount[3]. And so we must ask, "does the most common restraint, that of a three-point attached webbing seat belt with an emergency locking retractor, restrain motion and displacement sufficiently so as to prevent all injury?"

No, of course it doesn't. However, it does surprisingly well considering that the three point (lap/shoulder) seat belt is a design for which unobtrusiveness appears to have been a major design criterion. I say this because when one is *serious* about wearing a seat belt restraint, as for example, a racing car driver is serious, then a proper four or five point seat belt restraint is chosen and that is what is required by the authorizing racing associations. See figure 52.

Why then do we use three point restraint systems as the most commonly available webbing restraint system if it is not the best system? After all, four point and five point systems are better (i.e., four point and five point systems also greatly reduce the chance of "submarining" beneath the lap belt portion, such submarining causing terrible internal abdominal and spinal injuries). My answer is: "I don't really know; I have no idea who is responsible for this far reaching decision."

It would appear that someone (who?) presumed that the acceptability of seat belt restraints would be too greatly lessened if the somewhat more complex, somewhat more difficult to assume, and somewhat more expensive 4 point belt was offered.

But in fact, before mandatory usage of seat belts was legislated, only 15 percent or so of the population ever used these restraints at all, whether they were lap belts only or lap belt/chest harness (3 point) systems.

To state it bluntly, we made available, that is, we *required* the installation in all cars sold of a less-than-the-best system of restraints, the 3 point belts. Perhaps we had hopes that because it was simple to do, it would enjoy popular use. And when, despite prolonged educational programs, about 85 percent of car occupants still refused to wear the belts, we then made *mandatory* the use of the-less-than-the-best design by designating it as adequate to satisfy what we term our Federal Motor Vehicle Safety Standards.

As to fatality reduction, the conventional manual (i.e., non-automatic) 3 point restraint is estimated as 40 to 50 percent effective[4][5]. That sounds pretty good, but how can I know that I will be in the 40 or 50 percent that is effective?

And just what does "effective" mean?

Well, as used in the world of seat belt mavens, it means *"the reduction in fatalities, expressed as a percent, to a presently unbelted population that would result if all of its members were to use belts but not otherwise change their driving behavior[4]."*

And what does *that* mean? Well, *that* means that if there were say, 100 identical crashes and 20 unbelted occupants died, then had they all worn their seat belts, only 10 would have died and that would be termed as "50 percent effective." That's what "effectiveness" means. (Tell that to the ten that died with their seat belts on.) And that's what NHTSA means when it uses the term "effective" when it talks about reduction in fatalities due to a change in its regulations. (That's what NHTSA produces: regulations. Although NHTSA chooses to call its regulations "Federal Motor Vehicle Safety Standards," they definitely are not standards and some of them have not been safe.)

This isn't exactly new stuff. A 1973 paper by GM engineers estimated the lap/shoulder belt arrangement as 31 percent effective, as compared to say a lap belt at 17 percent effective, based on a detailed analysis of over 700 fatalities in 1967 to 1972 cars[6]. If anyone had even looked at a 1969 study of human volunteer subjects in test sled impacts comparing the flail of the human volunteers wearing only lap belts with that of human volunteers wear lap/shoulder harnesses, they could have seen the great differences in chest and head flail attributable to the presence of the torso restraint[7]. A year before the human test series, GM engineers had reported on seat belt design parameters, such as recommended attachment angles for webbing and belt loop length, and compared the lap belt restraint to a three point restraint in simulated 30 mph impacts using 2 different types of dummies[8]. Perhaps you can account for why it has taken more than 20 years since the earlier GM study and the combined USAF/NBS human volunteer study (and many similar, confirming studies since then) to require the replacement of rear seat lap belts with 3 point (lap/shoulder) belts. That utterly wasted 15 to 20 years translates to so many unnecessary deaths, and so many, too many, crippled lives.

I have no idea of the "effectiveness" of 4 or 5 point harnesses nor how many lives they could save, but I strongly believe that it would be many more because 4 point belts restrain the trunk from being thrown out of the chest harness in frontal crashes, when the principal direction of force is other than 12 o'clock, as is true of most frontal collisions' principal direction of force. To my knowledge, there are no comparative field studies between 3 and 4 point belts, nor of any usage differences documented between them. (Who, other than NHTSA, has the funds for such studies?) There are, however, studies which show less motion, which is to say, less displacement and less pathology at impact when 4 point belts are worn[9] [10].

For those of you desiring to briefly contemplate the long, slow history of car restraints, I suggest to you: *Historical perspective on seat belt restraint systems* by H.G. Johannessen, SAE paper 840392, 1984 and the 6 page "partial chronology" (appendix H) in the National Transportation Safety Board report NTSB/SS-86/03, available from the National Technical Information Service, Springfield, Virginia 22161, as PB86-917006. Johannessen's paper also provides helpful, simplified drawings of harness types, spool locking mechanisms and retractor assemblies.

RESTRAINT SYSTEM COMPONENTS

We speak of restraint *systems* advisedly. By itself, a harness of webbing attached to various parts of the car is not a restraint system: a webbing restraint harness is only a restraint harness made of webbing.

It has been found that the angle that the lap belt webbing forms with the floor of the vehicle, and the angle the attachment to the floor makes with regard to the occupant (as seen in plan view), and the angle of the seat pan itself, all are important determinants of the effectiveness of the seat belt harness[8][11]. These attributes are part of what we'd best call a seat belt restraint *system*, since a proper seat belt system has all these and a lot more components and aspects.

More components? More aspects? Well, yes. Clearly the elasticity of the webbing matters, as do the webbing attachment point locations, as does the fit of the webbing to the anthropometric needs of a given occupant, as does the spoolout of webbing on the spool (which is also altered by the amount of webbing still left on the spool when the belt is being worn), as does the width of the webbing, as does the amount of retraction pull on the webbing (which in part determines the amount of belt slack), as does the trigger for locking the belt (i.e., whether the belt locks because of webbing motion or because of vehicle motion), as does the lock being a spool lock or a lock on the webbing itself, as does the vehicle's crush characteristics, and so forth and so forth. The design of a seat belt restraint system is not nearly as simple as it appears to be.

Restraint system components should also include the padding within the vehicle, such as knee bolsters, as well as the energy-absorbing steering assembly. Some like to divide the components of restraint systems into *active* and *passive* components, depending on whether the component requires effort on behalf of the occupant, such as buckling a seat belt (active) or doesn't require the occupant to do anything, such as dash energy absorbing padding (passive). As a general rule safety experts advocate passive systems and components wherever possible.

Since there are so many aspects of the design of seat belt systems, how often do seat belts and their components fail?

A tidy field study of simple seat belt component failure (and of the adverse effects of both seat belts *per se* and of belt failures) is available in a Swiss study done in 1976[12], but most of those vehicles were European cars. It would be nice if someone else, say NHTSA, regularly did comparable studies in the United States.

However, from NHTSA's Fatal Accident Reporting System (FARS) we may derive incidental information by noting that, when seat belts were worn in fatal accidents, less than 2 percent of the victims were partially or fully ejected. Presumably, *any* form of ejection means that the seat belts failed mechanically, which then means that seat belts are mechanically operational at least 98 percent of the time, under crash conditions so severe as to cause the death of one or more of the occupants of the vehicle.

(That this is so 98 percent of the time *should* at the least be persuasive for those "seat belt defense" cases wherein the vehicles are disposed of before the case is filed, since a 98 percent probability of operationality should surely mean that a given seat belt system was operational "to a reasonable certainty."

However, there are some courts that demand, as an element of the seat belt defense, that seat belts can be considered as "operational" *only* if they were tested to be so in the specific vehicle involved, a requirement that surely cannot be met when the plaintiff had control of his vehicle and chose to scrap it before permitting the defendant access to inspect the vehicle! In effect, these courts have given the option that rightly is that of the defendant to the plaintiff, who then can deny the defendant access to the seat belt defense by destroying the vehicle. But then, Justice is blind, isn't it?)

INFANT AND CHILD RESTRAINTS

Child safety seats are classified into: infant, convertible, and toddler.

Infant seats - used from birth to about 1 year of age or 20 pounds, whichever comes first. As a rule they should be installed and used *only* in the rearward facing position.

Convertible seats - are used from birth to 40 pounds, (which is the mean weight for male children of age 4.5 years). Until the infant is developed sufficiently to easily hold up its head and to *sit up*, the seat should be installed rearward facing; thereafter it may be turned to face forward.

Toddler seats - are for children 20 to 60 pounds, (the latter being the mean weight for male children of about 8.5 years). Realistically, though, toddler seats rarely are used after 4 years of age. Most children and their parents use the seat belts, with or without cushion boosters, when they use anything at all.

How good are these infant and child restraints?

A study using only Volvo cars concluded that *rearward facing* child seats were 80 to 90 percent effective *with regard to injury reduction* (!) while the forward facing booster cushion/seats were 30 to 60 percent effective[13]. This study has especial merit since the car types were more comparable than usual in that they all were Volvos, but it has the confusion factor of *rearward facing* toddler *seats*, which appears unique to this study. Morbidity was not reported.

A 1987 study of the effects of child restraint usage laws on traffic fatalities in 11 states[14] agreed with previous similar studies, all of which have found about 30 percent effectiveness of child restraints with regard to injury reduction, but found *no reduction in fatalities attributable to child restraint usage*.

This lack of fatality response may well result from the variations in child fatality rates being so great in studies of the unbelted child that they would have to been at least 20 to 25 percent reductions to be statistically significant in restrained children. All of which tells us that child restraints appear to very substantially reduce crash injuries in children, but have not demonstrated fatality reduction. If there is fatality reduction attributable to child restraints, the reduction is something less than 20 to 25 percent.

A major problem of child restraints and a possible cause for their low apparent fatality reduction may be that they are so often misused, with a field-demonstrated misuse rate of 75 percent[15] as misrouting of the restraining belt or misuse (or absence of) the tethers necessary to anchor the restraints. Booster seats appeared to have an even greater rate of misuse in a pilot study[15].

You may also want to know that, according to the list sent to me by NHTSA's Office of Defects Investigation Enforcement and dated 1/13/92, there have been 198 separate recalls of infant and child "safety seats" representing untold millions of infant and child restraints.

I term these as "untold millions" since the NHTSA did not tell the number of restraints involved in each of these recalls. However, the largest child restraint recall I know of was for a defective buckle on 3 million Evenflo child restraints and covered a 5 year period of manufacturing by that vendor.

RESTRAINTS FOR CHILDREN OVER AGE FOUR: AN APPARENTLY EXPENDABLE GROUP

In chapter 2 I said that we seem to have largely given up on properly fitting restraints to millions of our citizens, which is to say that most restraints that fit adults don't fit well those under say, 16 years of age. And since seat belts are required only to fit the 5th to the 95th percentiles of adults, then about 10 percent of the adult population, or another 20 million or so adults may be added to 50 to 60 million children not fitted, for a grand total of about 75 million or so car occupants that are not clearly of great concern to NHTSA since restraint systems are not required to fit these persons.

At the time of this writing (1992), some 25 years since NHTSA was given its mandate, NHTSA requires for children under adult proportions that dynamic dummy tests be done utilizing only a 6-month-old sized dummy and a 3-year-old equivalent dummy.

Pray, what happens to kids from 4 to 17 years of age?

In fact the NHTSA has been in the child safety business for a while, having promulgated what it calls Safety Standards for "Child Restraint Systems," (FMVSS 213) under 49 CFR Ch. V, section 571.213, starting about 1980. Even that took 13 years to come about. But as they say, "there's been a lot of thunder but not much lightning." After all, NHTSA was created in 1966; how can it possibly have taken so many years to promulgate even such simple, inadequate regulations regarding child restraints?

Motor vehicle crashes have been the leading cause of death for American children under age 5[16] for as far back as I can remember, and this has not been changed in the more than 25 years since NHTSA came upon the scene.

In ref.[17] Dr. Koop (Surgeon General of the U.S. from 1981 to 1989, and a pediatrician by trade) reported that about 1,700 children die and another 170,000 are injured in motor vehicle crashes annually. The same reference noted that NHTSA claims that "proper use of existing child restraints could prevent 500 deaths and 56,000 injuries each year." Which I interpret to mean that *if* existing child restraints were used properly, then the best that NHTSA hopes for is about 30 percent effectiveness for current child restraints.

I think that we should be able to do a lot better than that.

In fact, I am sure that we could equal or surpass that, *even without child restraint systems*, just by requiring children under age 10 to sit in rear seats. And we could pick up even more "effectiveness" by requiring infant and child restraints to be used in rear seats only. I am sure of this because it has already been done elsewhere; in

France, for instance.

As noted by Partyka in 1984[18], "an unrestrained child in the back seat appeared to be about as safe as a restrained child in the front seat and a restrained child in the rear seat was safer still." Similar conclusions were reported earlier and elsewhere[19] as well as at an international meeting on the Biomechanics of Trauma in Children, *10* years earlier, in 1974[20][21].

In 1983 it was reported from France that children under age 10 were obliged *by law* to be only in the rear seats of cars[22]. *Quite simply, by requiring only that infants and children be placed in the rear seats of cars, our decreased morbidity and mortality from mandatory infant and child restraint usage laws in all 50 states probably were equaled or bettered by this simple but thoughtful French law*, a law which did not even require that anything be manufactured or bought. Of course, the French have gone on to specify and design infant and child restraints in addition to requiring their rear seat location. What an intelligent solution. How embarrassed we should be.

SEAT BELT SLACK AND THE "COMFORT AND CONVENIENCE FEATURE"

There have been a number of attempts to remove the slack from webbing restraints, ranging from inflatable webbing[3] to pyrotechnic and other webbing pretensionsers and webbing clamps[1] because *removing slack from the webbing reduces the flail volume*, and, expectantly, thereby reduces interior contact injuries. So I'll not dwell too long on a wholly inane effort instituted by our Big Three car manufacturers in the mid-1970's and lasting for more than 15 years which *deliberately increased seat belt slack*. The manufacturers' thesis appears to have been that by slackening the upper torso restraints more people would wear the restraints, which would then somehow make up for the fact that the restraints no longer worked as well (because of the added slack!). Think about that one for a while.

Barred in Europe, it was termed a "comfort and convenience feature" by the U.S. manufacturers. It was termed "the windowshade retractors" in the many law suits provoked by the reduced effectiveness of slack restraint webbing almost inevitably caused by these windowshade retractors. While I don't know exactly how much comfort and convenience it provided, a number of papers[23][24] showed that this feature enhanced injury production.

NHTSA rightly tried to bar the use of these so-called "comfort and convenience retractors,'' but withdrew its 1976 and 1979 "Notices of Proposed Rulemaking'' under what has been reported as considerable pressure from car manufacturers. Despite overwhelming argument by tests, professional publications, consumer groups, the insurance industry, as well as a growing number of lost litigations on this issue, the U.S. car manufacturers persisted and insisted on using this stupid device for more than 10 years, causing immeasurable enhancement of injuries in seat belt restrained occupants until the retractors were "voluntarily'' discontinued in the new models of 1989.

I guess that this just shows that we cannot rely on manufacturers to be the sole source of safety improvements, especially in restraint systems.

AUTOMATIC RESTRAINTS AND AIR BAGS

For reasons that you are probably familiar with and which I believe to be too foolish for me to go into, NHTSA currently offers car manufacturers the option of providing *either* automatic seat belt restraints *or* airbags with manual 3 point seat belts in order to meet the Federal requirement that 1990 and later cars be progressively equipped with "automatic restraints.''

Early reports utilizing the Fatal Accident Reporting System for 1985 to 1991 cars equipped with air bags (drivers' side) have shown statistically reliable and interesting results, of which ref.[25] is typical:

- compared to comparable cars equipped only with manual seat belts, adding air bags reduced fatalities an additional 28 percent;
- the reduction was greater in large cars (50 percent) than in midsized cars (19 percent) or in small cars (14 percent).

The great difference in efficacy of air bags between large cars and small cars again raises the question of whether 1) large cars provided more flail space, 2) large cars provided better crush characteristics, or 3) large cars have less intrusion into the occupant's flail volume. In chapter 2, figure 4 we found there was little or no relationship between flail distances and vehicle weight, which then leaves us with the conclusion that heavier cars have better crush characteristics and less occupant compartment intrusion.

We can say it once again: Grandpa was right: "Large cars are safer than small cars.'' And to this we can now add: air bags plus manual belts are better than just manual belts.

Since the car manufacturers now have the choice of providing either air bags plus manual seat belts or providing automatic belt cars, one must wonder whether this choice is truly an equal choice: are automatic belts the safety equivalent of an air bag plus manual belts?

Not according to a recent Highway Loss Data Institute special report they're not[26]. Using a survey of insurance claims information on both injury and inpatient hospitalization of drivers of 1990 cars with either air bags or automatic belts, the survey found (after standardizing the data) that air bag equipped car drivers had the same frequency of injuries as did the drivers of automatic belt cars, but the air bag car drivers were about 25 percent less liable to have received hospital treatment for their injuries. "Moderate" and "severe" injury rates were also about 28 percent less for drivers of air bag cars than for drivers of automatic belt cars. All of which seems to say that air bag car drivers involved with crashes will sustain the same rate of injury as do the automatic belt car drivers, but the automatic belt car driver will sustain more serious injuries, on the average.

Finally, because life has shown us little enough that is pure goodness, because there seems to be little Yin without some Yang, we had better ask if seat belt restraints and air bags can do harm as well as do good. That is, can air bags and seat belt harnesses themselves cause injuries?

To that question: as regards seat belts the answer is "yes", but the answer is *always* preceded by a statement to the effect that "there is little question but that seat belts do far more good than harm".

As regards air bags, the answer is "Of course". While it is true that a host of questions were raised as to the injury potential of air bags[27][28][29], the real world of crash events has not supported significant injuries as a result of air bag deployment, and has supported significant survival enhancement and injury reduction as a result of air bag deployment[25][30].

SEAT BELT INJURIES

Major reviews of seat belt induced injuries in automobiles have been published in 1968, 1970 and 1976[9][31][32], summarizing about 80-plus different injuries associated with seat belt use, many of them being fatal and all of them being unpleasant at best. However, since studies of seat belt effectiveness (supra) have invariably shown positive figures, ranging from about 20 percent to 80 percent effectiveness, depending on the particular restraint system used, there seems little question that seat belt re-straints clearly do very much more good than the harm that they cause, despite both the severity of some seat belt injuries and the diversity of available restraint systems that cause injuries.

Given the variety of injuries attributable to restraint systems even a cursory analysis of the injury mechanisms leaves little question but that there is room for considerable improvement in the design of restraints.

One obvious area begging for improvement is the fit of the diagonal webbing resulting in contact with an occupant's neck. When the diagonal belt is in contact with the antero-lateral aspect of the neck, as it is so often in children, young adults and short persons, it is not surprising that there are reports of cervical spine, cervical spinal cord and cervical vascular injuries[32]. Of course, simply providing a movable attachment point for the retractor of the D ring obviates this problem. Important too is the tendency for occupants whose necks are irritated by these anthropometric maldesigns to displace the offending webbing from the shoulder where it should be to an underarm location where it shouldn't be, for the under arm location has been shown to have high potential to kill[33].

Lap belt maldesign has been shown to cause submarining below the lap belt, often producing severe damage to both solid and hollow viscus as well as fractures and fracture dislocations of the vertebral column and damage to its contents[34].

The major and nearly singular source of information about specific seat belt in-duced injuries long has been case reports from clinical journals. However, it would seem that a governmental organization that brings about compulsory use of restraints then has not just a moral obligation, but has an absolute *duty* to study the causality of injuries that may be caused by seat belt use *per se* or caused by maldesign of the restraints that citizens are obliged to use. Canada has met this duty with a special task force to study seat belt induced injuries; the U.S. has not done so, and we should.

Reading this chapter concerned with restraint systems may well give the impres-sion that I am somehow dissatisfied with what I believe to have been unconscionably slow decision making by the NHTSA.

It is true; I am terribly discontented with that agency.

I am disheartened that, for example, it literally took an act of Congress to force NHTSA to require front-end air bags in all new vehicles (as of Sept., 1998). That's more than 25 years after air bags had proven their worth.

It's also more than 25 years since NHTSA was formed and there *still* exists no standard to match bumper heights between cars, vans, pickups and trucks.

(Even as I write this I am consulting in a case in which 3 children were killed in the rear seat of a vehicle struck in the rear by another passenger vehicle. Incredibly, although both vehicles shared the same manufacturer, the bumpers were of markedly different heights! The striking vehicle's bumper far overrode the struck vehicle, so that the striking vehicle never engaged the frame of the vehicle it struck; it simply pushed through the thin sheet metal of the trunk of the vehicle it struck and pushed the 3 children occupying the rear seat forward, crushing them against their parents in the front seats, killing all 3 children and badly injuring their parents.)

My discontent with the NHTSA originated in one emergency room or another. That's where I dealt with large numbers of unnecessarily mangled bodies and lives. I believe that at those very same moments, about 10 miles from my last emergency room in Maryland, the folks over at NHTSA were dealing only with large numbers. And the numbers didn't bleed, and clearly, they created no urgency over there.

It is true that there are competent and responsible members of the NHTSA. I know of many. Certainly, if blame is ever put at anyone's doorstep, it should be put precisely at the doorstep of those appointees and administrators who have followed our Capital's philosophy of loyalty to whoever appointed them, rather than following their own consciences, their own awareness that delays in this arena surely are paid for with blood.

Believe me; we *still* pay with blood each day for that agency's nonfeasance.

BIBLIOGRAPHY

1. Mitzkus, J.E. and H. Eyerainer: Three-point belt improvements for increased occupant protection. *SAE* paper 840395, 1984.
2. Dance, M. and B. Enserink: Safety performance evaluation of seat belt retractors. *SAE* paper 790680, 1979.
3. Dejeammes, M., Biard, R. and Y. Derrien: The three point belt restraint: investigation of comfort needs, evaluation of efficacy improvements. *SAE* paper 840333, 1984.
4. Evans, L.: Fatality risk reduction from safety belt use. *J Trauma* 27:746, 1987.
5. Partyka, S.C.: Lives saved by seat belts from 1983 through 1987. *DOT HS 807 324* (NHTSA, DOT), 1987.
6. Wilson, R.A. and C.M. Savage: Restraint system effectiveness - a study of fatal accidents. *SAE Safety Eng Seminar*, p. 27, June 1973.
7. Armstrong, R.W. and H.P. Waters: Testing programs and research on restraint systems. *SAE* paper 690247, 1969.
8. Louton, J.C. and T.W. Ruster: Restraint systems, design and performance parameters. *Proc GM Auto Safety Seminar*, Mich., July, 1968.
9. Snyder, R.G., Snow, C.C., Young, J.W., Crosby, W.M. and G.T. Price: Pathology of trauma attributed to restraint systems in systems in crash impacts. *Aerospace Med,* p. 812, Aug. 1968.
10. Stapp, J.P.: Part II. Effects of seat belts: man. *Env Biol*, p. 229, Fed Am Soc Exp Biol, Bethesda, 1966.
11. Leung, Y.C., Terriere, C., Fayon, A., Mairesse, P. and P. Banzet: An anti-submarining scale determined from theoretical and experimental studies using three-dimensional geometric definition of the lap-belt. *SAE* paper 811020, 1981.
12. Niederer, P., Walz, F. and U. Zollinger: Adverse effects of seat belts and causes of seat belt failures in severe car accidents in Switzerland during 1976. *SAE* paper 770916, 1977.
13. Carlsson, G., Norin, H. and L. Ysander: Rearward facing child seat - the safest car restraint for children? *33rd Ann Proc AAAM,* p. 249, 1989.
14. Wagenaar, A.C., Webster, D.W. and R.G. Maybee: Effects of child restraint laws on traffic fatalities in eleven states. *J Trauma 27:*726, 1987.
15. Shelness, A. and J. Jewett: Observed misuse of child restraints. *SAE* paper 831665, 1983.

16. *Injury in America*. Nat Acad Press, Wash., D.C., 1985.
17. Koop, C.E.: as reported in *Automotive Eng 100*:65, April 1992.
18. Partyka, S.: Papers on child restraints - effectiveness and use. *DOT HS 807 286*, June 1986.
19. Williams, A.F. and P. Zador: Injuries to children in automobiles in relation to seating location and restraint use. *Accid Anal Prev 9*:69, 1977.
20. Lowne, R.W.: Injuries to children involved in road accidents. *Proc Intl Mtg on Biomech of Trauma in Children*, p. 19, IRCOBI, 1974.
21. Ashton, S.J., Mackay, G.M. and P.F. Gloyns: Trauma to children as car occupants. *ibid*. p. 83.
22. Tarriere, C., Thomas, C., Brun-Cassan, F., Got, C. and A. Patel: From three year olds to adult size - how to ensure child protection in automobile accidents. *SAE* paper 831664, 1983.
23. Performance of lap/shoulder belts in 167 motor vehicle crashes. *vol 1, PB88-917002*, NTSB/SS-88/02, Washington, D.C., 1988.
24. Reichert, J.K. and T.J. Bowden: A study to determine the quantitative effects of seat belt slack. *Defense and Civil Institute of Environmental Medicine Report 80-R-64*, DOT, Canada, 1980.
25. Zador, P. and M.A. Ciccone: Driver fatalities in frontal impacts: comparisons between cars with air bags and manual belts. *IIHS*, Oct., 1991.
26. Driver injury experience in 1990 models equipped with air bags or automatic belts. *Insurance Special Report A-38*, Oct., 1991.
27. Patrick, L.M. and G.W. Nyquist: Airbag effects on the out-of-position child. *SAE* paper 720442, 1974.
28. Richter II, H.J., Stalnaker, R.L. and J.E. Pugh, Jr.: Otologic hazards of airbag restraint system. *SAE* paper 741185, 1974.
29. Mertz, J.H., Driscoll, G.D., Lenox, J.B., Nyquist, G.W. and D.A. Weber: Responses of animals exposed to deployment of various passenger inflatable restraint system concepts for a variety of collision severities and animal positions. *SAE* paper 826047, 1982.
30. Evans, L.: Airbag effectiveness in preventing fatalities predicted according to type of crash, driver age, and blood alcohol concentration. *32rd Ann Proc AAAM*, p. 307, 1989.
31. Snyder, R.G.: The seat belt as a cause of injury. *Marquette Law Rev 53*:211, 1970.
32. Sims, J.K., Ebisu, R.J., Wong, R.K.M., and L.M.F. Wong: Automobile accident occupant injuries. *JCEP 5*:796, 1976.

33. States, J.D., Huelke, D.F., Dance, M. and R.N. Green: Fatal injuries caused by underarm use of shoulder belts. *J Trauma 27*:740, 1987.

34. Ritchie, W.P., Ersek, R.A., Bunch, W.L. and R.L. Simmons: Combined visceral and vertebral injuries from lap type seat belts. *Surg Gynecol Obstet*, p. 431, Sept., 1970.

CHAPTER 11

INJURY MEASUREMENT SCALES

INTRODUCTION

This chapter is about the different ways we measure how much an occupant of a crashed vehicle has been broken and torn by the crash.

It is also about how we attempt to measure the long term consequences of breaking and tearing different parts of people.

In other words, this chapter is about with how we try to keep score. We would like to determine if we are doing better or doing worse at breaking and tearing people in crashes.

The specifics of **how we measure injury is critical to our assessment of crashworthiness, and unless we understand well what it is that we are measuring, such assessment can mislead and misdirect our efforts**.

We will try to distinguish the different things we are trying to measure so that we may better understand that an injury evaluated and quantified from the viewpoint of say, the cost of treating an injury, may have nothing at all to do with the injury measured from other viewpoints, such as its medical importance as an immediate threat to life, or an injury's potential for long term impairment, or its consequences as a disability in terms of diminished lifetime earnings.

An example of what may be wrong with how we usually measure crash injuries (that is, by using the Abbreviated Injury Scale) would be that of a scale giving equal value (AIS 2, "moderate injury") to a closed fracture of the heel and to a closed displaced nasal bone fracture. While they share the same low threat-to-life, they share nothing else in terms of impairment, cost of treatment, workmens' compensation or anything else.

Lest you are tempted to skip this chapter, let it be known that we have already entered a time epoch in medical/legal/insurance history in which *all injuries and illnesses are currently being measured in one or another quanta of severity*[1]. All diagnoses and treatments reimbursed by third part insurers are coded in a number of codes, such as the ICD-9 (the International Classification of Diseases).

Our simple expectation for severity injury scales is that severity injury software will be developed that will allow our uniquitous computers to whistle, hum, bark, and then cough up a severity score that is assigned to a particular patient. The score then will tell 1) the probability of that patient dying, 2) how much it will (probably) cost to treat that patient, 3) anything else that you can correlate and program, such as the probability of disability, of future illnesses, of changes in probable life-span and so forth.

All of this is true. But it is only partly true.

If the readers of this book are all adults, they have already learned that partial truths can kill you. While it is true that the severity scores can do what is listed in 1, 2, and 3, they cannot do it for any *one individual in particular*. That is, they can for example, tell us that *3 out of 4* times we may expect that the injuries sustained in a crash by a particular patient will cause his death. In fact, we know that *this individual* can only die once, not 3 out of 4 times. We can therefore only say that he is *liable* to die of his injuries, not that he *will* die of the injuries. What we are doing is making estimates that we call probabilities because we have created a mathematical process to create them.

Severity scores provide the basis for a computer probability that a certain sized group of patients with the correlated severity indices will fit computed predictions (with a considerably less than 100 percent fit).

Please don't get me wrong; I think such efforts are useful, important, and will get better with experience. I further believe that they will not be terribly accurate for a good number of years, probably not within my lifetime. You should never forget that a "probability" of an event happening is nothing more than a computed prediction. It is an elegant way of saying "an estimate." It is a mathematically derived guess which may or may not well describe a group response and which absolutely can neither describe nor predict an individual response.

When the numbers are large enough and the programs are sufficiently refined, the processed severity scores can suggest to us that a particular institution's record for treating, say, closed head injuries, is better or worse than the national average, or any other particular institution's record of treatment. In short, such programs may provide other cost and quality control information.

The largest of such efforts of which I am aware is under the sponsorship of the Health Care Financing Administration, and we will only mention some of its various versions, (termed "Medicare Mortality Predictor Systems"), such as APACHE (developed by George Washington University for intensive care patients), or AIM (Acuity Index Method), or CSI (Computer Severity Index), or Disease Staging, or

MedisGroups II, or PMC (Patient Management Categories).

Some of these systems utilize diagnoses, others use test and examination results, and some use both.

We will not deal further with the above systems for several reasons, not the least of which is that they are intended for anyone entering a hospital for any reason at all, from having a baby to having an appendix removed. We can do better than they can by limiting our scope to blunt trauma.

This chapter will be a small chapter. Like much of this book, it will not attempt to be encyclopedic, but rather will attempt to cover a lot of what I believe to be important crash injury territory. Important, that is, in that it will tell how and why we try to figure the "importance" of any one injury.

THE ABBREVIATED INJURY SCALE (AIS)

Of this scale it may be said (in the timeless phrase of Saddam Hussein), that the AIS is "the Mother of them all."

The AIS[2] was developed in the 1969 to 1971 period, under the sponsorship of the American Medical Association, the American Association for Automotive Medicine and the Society of Automotive Engineers. It followed some 20 years during which a variety of other injury measurement systems were used, none of which became well accepted. Of the early AIS, one of the contributors, J.D. States, was quoted[3] as saying:

> "Originally, three criteria were used to determine the AIS codes; energy dissipation, threat to life and permanent disability or impairment. As the AIS developed, and by 1977, threat to life became the principle criteria for coding. Energy dissipation was considered inappropriate for users other than vehicle designers. Disability has appeared to be too complex a criteria to incorporate in the AIS."

The AIS is a method of keeping a damage score by telling how bad the damage (injury) is. It does this by assigning to the damage a severity number (from the following severity number scale), *but note that this number doesn't tell you what was damaged*. As you will see shortly, the AIS 6-digit coding does locate the damage, but as we have seen, damage localizing coding is not what is used in most accidentology literature.

The AIS lacks any relationship between an AIS value and the cost of the injury or its impairment consequences. While the "severity" is coded, that single digit value disregards where in the body it occurs and the type of injury it represents. I earlier gave an example where a small tear in the rectum shares the same AIS value with a below the knee amputation, because they share the same "threat-of-life," but the impairment results are literally worlds apart. Here are what the AIS numbers represent:

AIS Number	Severity Code
1	Minor
2	Moderate
3	Serious
4	Severe
5	Critical
6	Virtually unsurvivable (Maximum injury in AIS 85)
9	Unknown

By the 1985 revision the AIS had learned to do what it can do and learned to do it very well. What the AIS does very well is estimate the degree of threat to life of any injury, and reduce such threat to a single digit number.

The single digit number applies to injuries within one of 9 general body regions, each of which has its own number. Two more numbers are then assigned to locating the organ or area and the next 2 digits are used to designate the severity level. A decimal then appears and, to the right of the decimal, the AIS severity code number. All of this results in a 6 digit code.

So what's the big deal about a 6 digit code?

Well, as we all should know by now, multi-digit codes are the stuff of which computer programs are made. *Thus the net result of the AIS is to provide a representation of the severity of (mostly blunt) injuries resulting from crashes in a form most easily processed by machines.* By correlating the AIS severity estimates with known subsequent outcomes, probabilities of outcomes were derived. That is the all and the only of what the AIS can and does do.

Because it was pretty clear on its face that someone with several AIS 4 (i.e., "severe") injuries was probably more liable to die that someone else with only a single AIS 4 injury, scales soon were developed to compensate for this deficiency of the AIS, such as the PODS (Probability of Death Score) and ISS (the Injury Severity

Score). The ISS survived as a score and the PODS didn't. The ISS soon had its own derivatives, developed to compensate for its own deficiencies.

THE INJURY SEVERITY SCORE (ISS)

The ISS was developed in 1974[4], about 3 years after the first AIS was published. It's developers included, among other notables, Dr. William Haddon, Jr., who had been the first administrator of the National Highway Safety Bureau (as NHTSA was then called).

The ISS is a single number, derived from the sum of the squares of the highest AIS grade in each of the 3 most severely injured body regions.

For a variety of reasons better discussed in ref.[5], the unmodified ISS should be used with caution and only as a very rough predictor of morbidity, mortality or disability, although for significant multiple injuries, it certainly is better than the AIS alone.

There have been other attempts to process multiple significant injuries with a single derived number because it is most convenient to process a single number, and you will see acronyms such as MAIS (which designates the most severe AIS injury), as well as OIC (an Occupant Injury Classification), OAIS, TR, and TRISS (a Trauma Score, which is a modification of an earlier Triage Index, combined with the ISS[6]).

A word or two about TRISS and its more recent developments is warranted. TRISS used *both* anatomic and physiologic indices of injury severity as well as patient age to derive a patient's probability of survival. TRISS was the basis of a new injury severity profile, the latest of which that I have found bears the acronym ASCOT (i.e., "A Severity Characterization of Trauma"), and combines values for the Glasgow Coma Scale, systolic blood pressure, respiratory rate, patient age and the AIS 85[7].

If you are wondering why I am burdening you with all this stuff about injury severity measurement systems, I am doing so to make a few important points to you:

1) that there are so many different systems of measuring injury severity and that they are still evolving should be eloquent proof to you that none of them is yet good enough to sufficiently predict what we wish we could predict: the final outcome of an injured person, including such items as disability, length of stay, resources required for proper treatment, etc., all as based on the initial assessment of his injuries, and

2) the more recent developments in injury scaling include physiologic indices of injury as well as anatomic indices, but the latter is the sole input of the AIS, and

3) indices such as sex, age and habitus are not yet included into most indices, also suggesting that their development has a way to go.

In short, there is good reason for you to be cautious in your reliance upon these injury indices and you may have the opportunity to have at those who do rely on these indices too heavily.

Now we will briefly look at the measurement of disability and the present quality of *its* predictability.

INJURY COST SCALES AND DISABILITY SCALES

As a general rule, (with all of the exceptions such general rules seem always to have), it appears to be perfectly obvious that **the greater the disability, the greater its cost, when such cost includes treatment, rehabilitation, lost wages and social security costs (i.e., society's disability costs).**

While there have been attempts to try to extract disability and long term impairment information from the AIS[8] [9], the early results showed just what you might expect: that a system designed to measure injury from the viewpoint of threat-to-life is a poor system for measuring injury from the viewpoint of disability.

The West Germans, bothered by a social cost for victim of road accidents estimated at about 30 *billion* dollars per year and convinced that further reductions in automotive crash morbidity and mortality would come about primarily "through improving the passive safety of motor vehicles[3]," developed what appears to me to be a first rate *cost related injury scale* to be used in addition to the AIS[3]. In reality, it is a comparative disability scale, since its base consisted only of a working (employed) population.

Utilizing statistics from the German Workmens' Compensation for 1985 (28 million employed persons between ages 15 and 65), as well as from 88,000 road accidents (causing 15,407 hospital treated victims, of which 6,170 suffered a reduction in gainful employment and 1,026 died), 2 injury cost scales were developed. One was for an Injury Cost Scale indexed to 100,000 DM for non-fatal injuries with societal costs, the second was for an Injury Cost Scale Lethal, similarly indexed to 100,000 DM for the societal costs of different fatalities. Clearly, these cost scales apply only to an employed population between ages 15 and 65.

Ignoring the costs as given in DM, the *indexed scales represent relative values*, thus permitting the identification of:

the most frequent injuries
the most severe injuries (as permanent impairment)
the most expensive injuries
the injuries with the highest rates of permanent impairment
as well as many other injury/cost factors.

The conclusions of these cost-related scales are so important and so useful to any reader of this book that I shall list them in the above order. (Percentages are rounded off to the nearest whole number.)

The Five Most Injured Body Regions (in-patients and fatalities)

1.	lower extremities	34 percent
2.	head	32 percent
3.	upper extremities	13 percent
4.	neck, spine	9 percent
5.	trunk	8 percent

The Ten Most Frequent Injuries (in-patients and fatalities)

1.	cerebral concussion	14 percent
2.	cerebral contusion	9 percent
3.	closed fracture of hip, pelvis, femur	7 percent
4.	closed fracture tibia/fibula	6 percent
5.	closed fracture foot	5 percent
6.	spine fracture	5 percent
7.	glenohumeral fracture	5 percent
8.	ribcage fracture	3 percent
9.	closed fracture radius/ulna	3 percent
10.	vertebral subluxation	3 percent

The Ten Most Expensive Single Injuries (without fatalities)
1. open skull fracture
2. closed hip joint fracture
3. open pelvis/femur fracture
4. open eye injury
5. closed skull fracture
6. thoracic spine fracture
7. cervical spine fracture
8. open lower leg fracture
9. open radius/ulna fracture
10. hip or thigh laceration

The Rates of Permanent Impairment for Different Injuries
(in decreasing order of importance)
1. fractured heel
2. eye injury
3. open fracture of femoral shaft
4. closed fracture of hip joint
5. open skull fracture
6. closed fracture of femoral neck
7. open fracture of pelvis/femur
8. closed fracture of head of tibia
9. open dislocation of knee
10. open fracture of shaft of tibia/fibula

I have employed what for me is an unusual amount of restraint in waiting until these lists were finished before suggesting that you please again note that, as mentioned earlier: a) extremities are the most injured body region, b) upper extremities (for which we have previously found that almost no NHTSA or SAE publications concern themselves) are the *3rd* most common car crash injury, c) 5 of the 10 most expensive injuries are of the extremities, and d) 8 of the 10 highest permanent impairment-rating injuries are of the extremities. Perhaps we ought to hold *some* concern for how extremity injuries come about.

PUTTING IT ALL TOGETHER; OR, WHAT HAPPENS WHEN WE RUB INJURY SCALES AGAINST EACH OTHER?

It is perfectly obvious (at least I think so) that the scales we use for measurement can alter what we think we measured. If we look at the world with infra-red sensors we would see a different world than that seen by visible light, or the world seen by x-ray sensors.

In the same way I could postulate a scenario where say, we make the use of restraint systems mandatory, thus increasing utilization rates from the 15 percent of the mid-1980s to the near 50 percent of the early 1990s. I could also posit that when restraints are not used, drivers in frontal collisions sustain severe lacerations and contusions of their chest, face and head (AIS 3,4,5).

If I then posit that when the usage of restraints increased, the restrained drivers' most common injuries changed from severe facial lacerations from striking the windshield to more severe facial fractures (especially LeFort II and III fractures) and to an increase in closed head injuries with increased residual neurologic deficits, because the restrained drivers now struck the steering wheel with their heads and faces, *but we still recorded only AIS 3,4,5.*

Although the AIS values stayed the same, the societal cost increased greatly, as the number of disabling closed head injuries and long term impairments increased many fold.

While all of the above is only a postulated scenario, how in the world would we know if it *was* real?

The AIS would not necessarily reflect it. That's one of the problems that I have, not with the AIS (which is a fine severity scale of the threat-to-life persuasion), but with *the inappropriateness of using the AIS scale exclusively for the assessment of crash injuries in most reports concerned with crash.*

As I have said before, the Fatal Accident Reporting System does well enough for threat-to-life at AIS 6 (fatal). Non-fatal injuries are better described when they are described, and better measured by other measures, such as societal costs, impairment, disability, and so forth.

It is perfectly obvious (at least I think so) that injury scales derived purely from the viewpoint of threat-to-life are best for "triage" purposes.

What is triage? Why, triage is an exercise in setting medical treatment priorities, such priorities being three in number:

1) those who *probably* will not survive, even with medical treatment;
2) those who *probably* will recover, even without treatment; and
3) those who *probably* need treatment in order to survive.

Triage is generally saved for situations in which a large number of casualties exist, such casualties being larger than medical facilities could immediately treat. Casualties will be triaged (that's a French word for "sorted") into the three groups listed above and group 3 would be treated first.

Triage is what I believe to be the primary rational reason behind trauma scales such as ISS, TRISS and later derivations. Having spent some time in emergency rooms, I know that times are not rare when there are more patients than treating staff. We used "triage nurses" to first evaluate patients when we were too busy for anything else.

What I have difficulty understanding is why in the world the Abbreviated Injury Scale, which in essence is a triage scale, is applied to and is used in the field of crash injury causation.

Except for triage (and I suppose quality of care evaluation too) I can think of no good reason to even be interested in a threat-to-life scale if your business is making cars and roads safer.

There is no way for a reader to go from a reported AIS number to what was injured, how the injury came about and what residual impairment resulted.

What NHTSA should be concerned with is fatality production and impairment production and the *specific* causes of each in accidents. It is the utter lack of specificity implicit in the AIS reporting that made it difficult for me to find data for the title subject of this book, and the title subject, it seems to me, is the very essence of NHTSA's mandate.

Perhaps more appropriate to the NHTSA mission, and to your interests, since you have bothered to read this book, would be the concept of A.C. Malliaris, the concept of "harm," defined as "the sum of injuries of crash victims, with each injury weighted in proportion to the economic cost of the outcome of such injury whether fatal or not[10]," discussed earlier in this book. Since other authors, also from the NHTSA, have also utilized the harm concept[11], the approach should not be news to NHTSA, particularly since it was published at least 10 years before this book was written[12] and represents a thoughtful and appropriate injury index for what NHTSA should be doing.

And at least as appropriate to the NHTSA mission also are the splendid disability scales (ICS and ICSL), relatively recently developed by the Institute for Forensic Medicine at Mainz and the German Workmens' Compensation at St. Augustin, published in this country by the AAAM[3]. Let us hope that the ICS and the ICSL will soon have numbers assigned to their lists of "body region and type of injury", so that the computer mavens can put together the AIS and the ICSs.

But to reduce injuries and deaths *it is most appropriate to first establish exactly how the injuries occurred, including available, retrievable information characterizing the accident (direction and magnitude of collision, etc.)* in conjunction with the information specifying and characterizing the injuries that occurred.

NHTSA, please report exactly what the injuries were as a result of a given crash. You can stop telling us that the injuries were "serious", because "serious" (AIS 3) is just about useless in determining the mechanism of quite how the "serious" injury came about. We need to know what the injuries are, not that they were more or less serious as an estimated threat-to-life.

I know that I need and would use such long-overdue information for crash injury causation analysis.

I believe that designers of cars could and should use such more specific information to bring about fatality and injury reduction.

How can vehicles be made safer without making available information as to what injuries are produced by what specific crash conditions and what the mechanism is for producing a specific injury?

I believe that litigation may be reduced as attorneys and insurers could better evaluate the validity of a claim. (Evaluating the validity of a claim, you see, requires an understanding of whether the specific injury(ies) claimed are proximately related to the accident event, and background data for such evaluation is simply not within the AIS.)

I believe that most of you who read this book hold a great and largely unfulfilled interest in such specific crash injury data, considering that you have just proven your interest in what happens to people-in-cars-that-crash by reaching this, the end of the next to the last chapter of this book.

BIBLIOGRAPHY

1. Gardner, E.: Measuring degrees of illness. *Mod Healthcare*, p. 22, Dec. 16, 1988.
2. *The Abbreviated Injury Scale.* 1985 rev. AAAM, Arlington Heights, 1985.
3. Zeidler, F., Pletschem, B., Mattern, B., Alt, B., Miksch, T., Eichendorf, W. and S. Reiss: Development of a new injury cost scale. *33rd Ann Proc AAAM*, p. 231, 1989.
4. Baker, S.P., O'Neill, B., Haddon, W.H. and W.B. Long: The injury severity score: a method for describing patients with multiple injuries and evaluating emergency care. *J Trauma 14*:187, 1974.
5. Copes, W.S., Champion, H.R., Sacco, W.J., Lawnick, M.M., Keast, S.L. and L.W. Bain: The injury score revisited. *J Trauma 28*:69, 1988.
6. Boyd, C.R., Tolson, M.A. and W.S. Copes: Evaluating trauma care: the TRISS method. *J Trauma 27*:370, 1987.
7. Champion, H.R., Copes, W.S., Sacco, W.J., Lawnick, M.M., Bain, L.W., Gann, D.S., Gennarelli, T., MacKenzie, E. and S. Schwaitberg: A new characterization of injury severity. *J Trauma 30*:539, 1990.
8. MacKenzie, E.J., Shapiro, S., Moody, M. and R. Smith: Predicting post-trauma functional disability for individuals without significant brain injury. *28th Ann Proc AAAM*, p. 173, 1984.
9. Hirsch, A.E. and R.H. Eppinger: Impairment scaling from the Abbreviated Injury Scale. *ibid.*, p. 209, 1984.
10. Malliaris, A.C., Hitchcock, R. and M. Hansen: Harm causation and ranking in car crashes. *SAE* paper 850090, 1985.
11. Digges, K.H., Roberts, V. and J. Morris: Residual injuries to occupants protected by restraint systems. *SAE* paper 891974, 1989.
12. Malliaris, A.C., Hitchcock, R. and J. Hedlund: A search for priorities in crash protection. *SAE* paper 820242, 1982.

CHAPTER 12

PATTERNS OF INJURY IN FRONTAL, LATERAL, REAR, AND ROLLOVER CRASHES

INTRODUCTION

This last chapter is another topic about which 4 books could be written.

In fact, one book has already been written: *Injuries Following Rear-End Automobile Collision*, by W.D. deGravelles, Jr. and J.H. Kelley, (published by Charles C Thomas, Springfield, 1969).

This last chapter is a brief overview of injury patterns for the different major types of collisions, either single or multivehicle. An overview of injury patterns may be all that is possible or even appropriate for a primer.

GENERAL

I recall a case in which 3 parolees, drunk and without drivers' licenses, missed a curve on a lonely far north country road and rolled a pickup truck. One occupant was rendered paraplegic while the other 2 sustained only trivial injuries. No one had worn seat belts and all of them denied that they were the driver. As is too often the case, the vehicle was promptly destroyed at a salvage yard and could not be inspected. Only a few inadequate photos of the vehicle (exterior only!) were taken at the scene after the accident.

Two of the occupants had injuries so typical of their location within the car and of the particular crash conditions that there was no difficulty getting 3 experts in injury causation to agree as to where each occupant had been located.

What also made this case more interesting than usual was the fact that the plaintiff's attorney did not tell any of the experts that there were others analyzing the case until after all 3 experts had been separately deposed, at which time I found that there were 2 other experts on the case and that we had all totally independently come to exactly the same conclusions as to where in the vehicle each occupant had to have been located.

Although I refer to such cases as "King Solomon" cases, they are more often than not relatively easy because, more often than not, the patterns of injury are characteristic of the occupants' location within the vehicle for a given crash direction as well as being characteristic of the use or non-use of restraints. Note that I have said "more often than not," and that I did not say "always."

As a general rule then, it may be said that **each principal direction of force (collision direction) has its own, rather typical constellation of injuries and each location within a particular vehicle also has a usual pattern of injuries**.

It may also be said that **the pattern of injuries sustained for a given principal direction of force and in a given location within a vehicle will often indicate whether or not seat belt restraints were being utilized by the occupant**.

While injury patterns often are typical and characteristic of location within a vehicle and of use or non-use of restraints, let me again emphasize the several factors we have previously mentioned as modifiers of injuries, such as sex, age, size and habitus of the victim. Along with these occupant attributes, vehicle characteristics such as stiffness and occupant flail space also are important determinants of what injuries will occur, of what patterns of injuries will result from a given direction and magnitude of crash and from a given location within the vehicle.

Let me add that in analyzing cases a working knowledge of the general mechanisms of injury causation, much of which has been given herein, is an absolute necessity and a minimum one at that.

Injuries that are not present often are as important as the injuries that are present. For example, the absence of road burns on an occupant ejected and found on the roadway tells us that the ejection was a terminal event. The ejected occupant *should have had* road burns. Therefore, the ejectee clearly had almost no remaining kinetic energy. He must have *fallen* from the vehicle after it had very nearly stopped moving, because had the occupant had residual velocity he would have rolled or slid after leaving the vehicle and would have had at least some, usually quite extensive road burns (i.e., skin abrasions characteristic of the abrasiveness and dirt content of a road's surface).

FRONTAL IMPACTS

The Driver

After I started this chapter, I received my copy of the 36th Annual Stapp Car Crash Conference Proceedings. In it I found a report about the somewhat uncommon topic of foot and ankle injuries. The report also included a good deal of information about belted and unbelted drivers' injuries and the parts of the cars that caused such injuries in frontal collisions[1], so we will use that report here.

The data comes from the Technical Accident Research Unit in Hannover, Germany, a multidisciplinary team that has diligently and continuously investigated traffic accidents since 1985 in an attempt to study vehicle and occupant crash kinematics, and I am comfortable with their data. (That means just that; I am comfortable with their data. It should not be taken to mean that I necessarily agree with their interpretation or with anyone else's interpretation of their data.)

Table 10 is derived from this study[1] and shows car components which caused injuries in frontal collisions for 253 unrestrained and 1141 restrained drivers.

TABLE 10

FRONTAL COLLISIONS AND VEHICLE COMPONENTS CAUSING INJURIES TO UNRESTRAINED AND RESTRAINED DRIVERS (after ref.[1])

Car Part Causing Injury	Unrestrained (n = 253) % Injured	Restrained (n = 1141) % Injured
Windshield	29 %	7 %
Dash (instrument panel)	20 %	16 %
Steering assembly	15 %	21 %
Seat belts	-	16 %
Side of vehicle	7 %	6 %
Floor of vehicle	8 %	8 %
Other parts	21 %	26 %

While we shall shortly discuss the differences in injury patterns between the driver and the right front passenger, certain questions are posed by this table, and let us at least ask them before we move on.

How do you suppose that 7 percent of the *restrained drivers* managed to strike the windshield despite having the steering assembly in front of them, between them and the windshield, in fact?

Even more remarkably, how did 16 percent of the *restrained drivers* manage to strike the dash board, despite wearing restraints and despite having the steering assembly in front of them? What part(s) of the drivers probably struck the dash board?

Why did more *restrained drivers* strike the steering assembly than did *unrestrained drivers*? What body parts did the *restrained drivers* hit against the steering assembly?

Again note (as we did in chapter 5) that there is no clear difference in the injury rate caused by floor pan buckling in the restrained versus the unrestrained driver. That is, injuries below the knees appear to occur with about the same frequency whether or not seat belt restraints are used[1] [2]. Finally, note that about 16 percent of the injuries sustained by restrained drivers were caused by the restraints themselves.

Injuries caused by restraints generally are not life threatening, most usually being fractures of the ribs underlying the restraint webbing, although an occasional sternal fracture will occur too. There also have been reported many other, often bizarre injuries caused by using restraints, ranging from ruptured gall bladders to decapitation. While such life threatening seat belt injuries are not absolute rarities, neither are they terribly common.

Restraint system induced injuries increase in number in direct proportion to increasing age[3] as well as to increasing delta v.

Driver Injury Patterns Compared to Right Front Occupant Injury Patterns In Frontal Crashes

Having compared what parts of vehicle interiors are struck by restrained drivers with those struck by unrestrained drivers, we will next look to a 1980 Canadian study in which 3 point belt restrained drivers' injury patterns are compared with similarly restrained right front occupants' injury patterns, for a number of frontal collisions[4].

TABLE 11

INJURY PATTERNS IN RESTRAINED DRIVERS AND RIGHT FRONT OCCUPANTS IN FRONTAL COLLISIONS (after ref.[4])

Body Region Injured	Driver	Right Front Occupant
Head/face	39 %	20 %
Neck	2 %	2 %
Shoulder/chest	22 %	23 %
Pelvis/abdomen	5 %	22 %
Upper extremities	11 %	14 %
Lower extremities	22 %	14 %
Other	-	5 %

While it is easily seen that restrained drivers injure their heads, faces and lower extremities about twice as often as do restrained right front passengers, and right front passengers injure their abdomen and pelvis more than 4 times as often as do restrained drivers, this information certainly doesn't provide a sufficient basis for inspecting an injury pattern and, from that inspection alone, declaring who was the driver and who was the right front passenger.

We'd best become a bit more precise before we can claim insight sufficient for "King Solomon" cases.

For example, "frontal impact" is not a sufficiently precise descriptor of the accident conditions from which these data were obtained. Reference[4] appears to have reached the same conclusion and therefore it divided frontal impacts into the Collision Deformation Classification adopted by the Society of Automotive Engineers as SAE J244.

This classification is an "SAE Recommended Practice" wherein frontal crash deformation, for instance, is divided into 5 possible regions and to the letter F (for Frontal) there is added R, C, L (obviously, for Right, Center and Left frontal) and the letters Y and Z for C + R and C + L, respectively. What results allows "FY" to represent a frontal right side and center area impact deformation. All of this is then added to a 7 character code, so that we end up with a rather large collision deformation code number. The resultant large number with upper case letters imbedded within it vaguely reminds me of a Vehicle Identification Number.

Anyway, the author correlated these frontal collision deformations with the Abbreviated Injury Scale numbers and, to my surprise, despite the diluted data input, there was produced some rather useful and arresting information:

1) two thirds of the frontal impacts were offset frontal collisions, the majority of which were *left* frontal offsets;

2) *drivers* sustained their most serious injuries when the impacts were *left* frontal offsets; (and, of course, the more severe the crush deformation, the more severe the injuries);

3) where the collision damage was offset to the right, *driver* injuries did not exceed AIS 2, which is to say they were "minor" or "moderate" under the AIS Severity Code (Abbreviated Injury Scale, 1985 revision);

4) about one-half of the injured right front occupants were injured in frontal collisions wherein there was no offset.

Now are we better equipped to decide what occupant sat where in given frontal collision? I believe so. For now we know that **offset impacts will preponderate in frontal collisions, and when offset, we know that the occupant on the struck offset side will usually incur the worst injuries**.

To the Table 11 information as to the commonness of certain injury clusters as they relate to location within the car we now will add the relative probable severity of injury clusters (patterns) as they relate to whether the frontal impact was central or offset, and to which side it was offset.

As also noted earlier in this book, offset frontal collisions are more common than frontal center ("distributed") collisions. In fact, **offset frontal collisions are about twice as common as frontal center distributed collisions** in this study[4].

(We may again wonder, as car manufacturers have done both frequently and vociferously, as to why collision tests required by NHTSA are the *least common*, pure frontal, distributed collisions).

Let us stop here for a moment and put together an example to help us to see how smart we have become:

Say we have 2 average size male 20 year old victims from a right frontal (right offset) crash of a sub-compact car with an average crush of 12 or 13 inches. Say that they both were wearing restraints, but both claim a loss of consciousness at the time of the accident and claim that they cannot remember who was driving. Say occupant "A" sustained a complex right ankle fracture, a contused forehead with 2 black eyes, but no other significant injury, although his left knee was contused.

Occupant "B" had no apparent injuries other than a claimed brief loss of consciousness and a sore mouth, with 2 broken teeth, bloody gum margins and swollen lips with lacerations inside of the lips. Both of his knees were contused too.

Who was driving? What are the bases for your conclusions?

(I suppose that I should provide answers to these questions at the end of this chapter rather than interrupt the flow of the text, but in truth, I have no stomach for such things. We will instead just briefly interrupt "the flow").

Who was driving? "B" was driving.

What are the bases for this conclusion? Let us look at each factor as it came up in the presentation of the example.

1) The occupants were of similar age, size and of the same sex; this means that there should be no differentiating effects attributable to these factors.

2) The crash was a *right* frontal offset crash of (very) approximately 20 mph delta v; (derived from multiplying the 13 inches of crush by 1.5), which means that: a) the right front passenger is in greater jeopardy of injury than the driver, and b) that there is, particularly in a small car, a greater risk of lower leg injury due to footwell intrusion on the right side rather than on the left side, and indeed, occupant A sustained just such an injury and occupant B did not. (Count 1 for A being the passenger and B the driver.)

3) Both occupants were said to be restrained, which more likely would keep the right front passenger from striking the windshield but would not keep him from striking the dash with his head, since the restrained occupant head would still have about a foot and a half of forward displacement despite the 3 point restraint system[5]. The dash board is a largely broad and smooth contact area, more likely to cause a contusion than a laceration. Bleeding in and beneath the forehead and anterior scalp from a contusion will commonly dissect down to the soft and distensible tissues of the eyelids, causing black eyes. (Count another one for A being the passenger, not the driver.)

4) Occupant B sustained broken teeth, and that should call up an image of a *hard* surface that was struck by the mouth, in contrast to that of the dash. From barrier crash tests we know that the *restrained* driver's head will strike either the hub or the rim of the steering wheel in the vast majority of frontal crashes[5], and a bloodied mouth with buccal surface lip lacerations and with broken teeth would not be an un-

common outcome of such contact. (You may also want to know that the delicate nasal bones are 3 or more times more often fractured in drivers'-head-to-steering-wheel contacts than are broken teeth or fractures of any of the other facial bones[6].)

More likely than not, "B" was the driver.

It also is common for both restrained front seat occupants to contact the dash with their knees[5] and here they both did just that.

And now, back to the text.

Typical unrestrained driver and right front seat occupant injuries in gross will follow the contacts and kinematics described in Chapter 1 and are illustrated in figure 1 of that chapter. Both unrestrained occupants' knees strike the dash about 60 milliseconds into the crash. The unrestrained driver then strikes the chest/abdomen into the steering assembly (at about 75 ms) and strikes and/or penetrates the windshield with the head/face at about 90 to 100 ms.

The unrestrained right front occupant strikes the dash with his chest/abdomen at very nearly the same time that his head/face strikes and/or penetrates the windshield, at about 90 or 100 milliseconds after the crash began.

Again in gross, the unrestrained driver and unrestrained right front seat passenger share injuries to the same three general areas: the head/face, the chest/abdomen and the knee/femur. However, as with restrained occupants, the principal direction of force and the specific vehicle flail volumes will generally provide sufficient additional information to allow for localization of occupants within the crashed vehicle.

Rear Seat Occupant Injury Patterns in Frontal Crashes

There are few reports on this subject. With regard to fatalities, the rear seat position in and of itself (i.e., independent of any restraints) appears to provide about a 25 to 30 percent fatality reduction as compared to either of the front seat locations (calculated from table 5, ref.[7]).

In his study of the interactions between car occupants during crash, Faerber[8] describes the unbelted rear occupant in a frontal crash as moving forward, striking the back of the front seat before him with his knees (at about 60 to 90 milliseconds) and with his thorax shortly afterward. He also noted that the design of front seatbacks generally does not significantly damp the knee and thorax impacts from the rear seat occupant. The front seat occupant therefore is rather fully loaded by the accelerated mass of the rear occupant or a portion of a rear occupant striking the front seat back.

In 3 of Faerber's tests the front seat adjustment failed under this increased loading, allowing the front seat to go forward. I can recall many accidents in which rear occupant loading of the front seat back caused the front seat occupant to be sandwiched between the loaded front seat back and the dash, thus causing dreadful crush injuries of the chest and abdomen, as you would expect.

When rear occupants were present in a frontal crash, I would urge that the seat back in front of them be carefully inspected. Incredibly, I have found seat backs made only of a metal frame and a sheet of soft foam with a thin vinyl cover, all of which has the ability to attenuate a blow to the seat back about equal to a dish cloth draped over the metal frame. This is most commonly found in off-road vehicle seat backs. I also recall a luxury passenger car wherein the front seat backs had a surprisingly thick, flat metal plate at the rear seat side of the front seat passenger seat back. This plate surely provided protection for the front seat occupants' backs, and, as a rigid plate, surely would also provide a way to break the knee caps or the femoral condyles of the rear seat occupants, or harm whatever body parts that struck them.

If one measures the flail space allowed a rear seat occupant and then also measures the occupant displacements that are known to occur despite the use of restraints[5], rarely will you find sufficient flail space provided the rear occupant that would prevent a rear occupant from striking the seat in front of him with *some* part of his body, whether it is an extremity, head or chest. And I have yet to find a single passenger car which has provided adequate padding in anticipation of this crash contact.

LATERAL (SIDE) IMPACTS

Of the passenger vehicles involved in multivehicle fatal crashes in the U.K. in 1990, 30 percent were lateral or side crashes, about evenly divided between the right and left sides of the struck vehicle[9]. This corresponds quite well with that reported for Germany in 1980 (also about 30 percent)[8], and in the U.S., as reported in NHTSA's Fatal Accident Reporting System for 1990. In other words, for multivehicle crashes, about 1 of every 3 passenger vehicle death results from side impacts.

Most multivehicle side impacts occur at intersections, which tells us[10] that:

1) most side impacts are from vehicles traveling essentially perpendicular to each other,
2) the struck car generally is traveling more slowly than the car that strikes it;
3) the struck car generally has a low delta v (velocity change);
4) the time epoch for the side collision is only slightly greater than that of a frontal collision, which is to say that side collisions also take place over a period of about 100 milliseconds.

As you might expect, because the sides of a vehicle have very much less room and less structure as compared to the front or to the rear of a car, in a lateral collision the vehicle structures intrude into the passenger compartments more readily, more often and more severely than they do in frontal or rear collisions of equivalent delta v. Intrusion is a major cause or a contributing cause to most "same side" (struck side) collision injuries.

Additional injuries are caused when the struck car is accelerated at right angles to its initial travel, inertially compelling the struck side occupant to strike his head on the (currently unpadded) struck side of the car while causing the far side occupants to be inertially thrown toward the struck side of the car, to impact with other occupants and with the car's interior[10]. A detailed analysis of the acceleration, velocity and displacement time histories of the impacted vehicle, its door and the same side occupant's chest is given in ref.[10], which also reviews occupant kinematics in side collisions.

Until the mid-1970s little apparent attention was paid to lateral collisions, either in the open literature or by our National Highway Traffic Safety Administration. The reasons for this have eluded me. However, I am pleased to report that, for whatever reason, the mid-1970s saw a sudden surge of research and interest in side collisions which has culminated in new requirements and tests for side impact protection.

The Federal Motor Vehicle Safety Standards for side impact protection (571.214) have been an embarrassment. They allow for the *least* side impact protection to be provided for the *smallest* vehicles, the smaller vehicles obviously needing such protection the most. (Can you imagine that? As I sit here today and write about it, the so-called "Safety Standard" still in effect insists that the smaller the vehicle, the less side door strength is required.) I'll not dwell further on our past idiocy except to say that from late 1993 onward, more demanding dynamic side impact tests will be required, encompassing all passenger vehicles by 1996.

However, for reasons also unclear to me, *far side occupants are not involved in the new side collision test procedures, nor are head injuries covered by the new side impact "standard".*

Please note that while far side occupants have nearly the same death rate as near side occupants, the *far side occupants are most liable to die from a head injury*, and are about 30 percent more liable to die from a head injury than are same side occupants. Head injuries are also the leading cause of death for same side occupants[9].

Since head injury is the most common cause of death in side impacts, why are head impacts not to be measured? Perhaps head impacts are not to be measured in side impacts because they are difficult to measure; or perhaps if measured, they may too often be found unacceptably high. Or perhaps, as a dear friend has often said, there never was a public problem so difficult to solve that it could not be completely ignored by the agency responsible for solving it.

It is worth distinguishing lateral impact injury patterns into those that occur to occupants on the struck side (also called the "near side, same side, or the impact side") from those that occur to occupants on the opposite side ("far side"), one reason being that they have different patterns of injury[9], and another reason being that, *for struck side occupants, restraints may be more of a sword than a shield.* That is, there is (controversial) evidence that *struck side occupants wearing restraints are more liable to die and are more liable to have severe injuries than are unrestrained struck side occupants*[9][11]. (The authors of ref.[9] do not state this attribute of seat belts in lateral collisions, but in table 1, page 3 of ref.[9], that's what their data show.)

Adverse effects of seat belts are most evident in small cars and at higher delta v's, say greater than 20 mph. Thus the increase in deaths and injuries to restrained same side occupants increases with increasing intrusion; a not unpredictable outcome for an occupant held in place by restraints as a portion of the car attempts to occupy the same space.

Lateral Collision Injury Patterns

The injuries caused to same side occupants that are attributable to intrusion and to the occupants' inertial displacement to the struck side are essentially the same for front seat and rear seat occupants. These characteristic injuries are seen in table 12, derived from ref.[9].

TABLE 12

"SERIOUS"-TO-FATAL INJURIES BY BODY REGION FOR FATALITIES IN STRUCK SIDE AND OPPOSITE SIDE CRASHES

Injury Site	Struck Side	Opposite Side	Injury Source*
Head	64 %	82 %	vehicle side interior
Neck	12 %	20 %	vehicle side interior
Chest	85 %	73 %	door/side structure
Extremities	23 %	22 %	(not noted)
Abdomen	59 %	49 %	door/side structure
Pelvis	26 %	14 %	door/side structure

*(Indicates that these sources are the cause of more than half of the injuries at each site.)

There were no differences noted between restrained and unrestrained occupants in this particular study either for struck side or opposite side occupants, except for an increase in head injuries for opposite side unbelted occupant head injuries, which were a third more common than for restrained opposite side occupants.

The authors believed almost half of the side impact deaths in this study were preventable by stronger side structures and padding[9].

(Since we have just entered into the realm of prevention and future design considerations for side impacts, I should mention an interesting and useful paper by Daniel[12], which I commend to you for both its lateral impact time histories and for its presentation of potential design improvements in vehicle structures to reduce injury and death from lateral impacts.)

Before leaving side impacts, we should appreciate that, as emphasized by Careme[10], *the forward velocity of the struck vehicle is an important factor in causing the injuries sustained by far side occupants*:

1) right front passengers in left side collisions strike the dash panel most frequently;
2) drivers in right side collisions strike the steering assembly most frequently.

Finally, as a last word before leaving side impacts, let me remind you that **the design of 3 point seat belts permits most restrained far side occupants to be thrown out of the** torso portion of their seat belts as a result of side impacts. *In lateral collisions, 3 point seat belt restrained far side occupants should therefore be considered as (functionally) restrained only by lap belts.*

REAR COLLISIONS

If we consider multivehicle collision fatalities, then rear impacts (5, 6 and 7 o'clock) caused 11.6 percent of car occupant deaths in 1985 and only about half that rate (6.7 percent) 5 years later, in 1990, both rates according to the Fatal Accident Reporting System reports for those years. Whether this means that our brakes are getting better or that our vehicles now have less aggressive front-end structures or that we have become more attentive to our driving, or that the NHTSA has changed what directions it counts as rear impact is not known to me.

Suffice it to say that from 5 to 10 percent of multivehicle crash deaths are due to rear end collisions. More modern statistics (which may be using more "modern" definitions of what constitutes a rear collision) suggest that rear collisions cause 3.5 percent of fatalities, 7.6 percent of serious injuries and almost a quarter of all car injuries[13].

In 1974, using a variety of data bases at the University of Michigan, Huelke and Marsh[14] found a number of interesting attributes of rear end collisions:

1) one-fourth of all collisions are rear end collisions, but
2) rear end crashes represent less than 4 percent of crash fatalities.
3) In urban areas, rear end crashes are 5 times more common than in rural areas, and
4) in urban areas rear end collisions are 5 times as common as frontal collisions (!).
5) Rear end collision fatalities are more common in rural than urban areas.
6) Neck injury is 3 to 5 times more frequent than any other body region.
7) Neck injury frequency does *not* increase with increasing rear end crush.
8) Neck injury is about 10 percent more frequent in females.

According to Tarriere[15], about one in five car occupants involved in rear collisions complain of neck pain as a subjective syndrome (i.e., AIS = 1). That's about the same occurence as in lateral collisions and about twice as common as in frontal collisions.

In a 1988 report by Lovsund et al[16] about 10 percent of occupants of rear end collisions sustained neck injuries. That study, incidentally, credited head restraints (head rests) as being "approximately 30 percent" effective.

Even though most rear end collision neck injuries rate "only" as an AIS 1, or "minor injury," *one-third of all injuries with permanent disability are neck injuries, which is the most common injury of rear end collisions*[16].

In a study of rear impacts which utilized 6 unembalmed, 3-point restrained cadavers, and the Daisy Decelerator Sled at Holloman AFB, Alamogordo, New Mexico[17], delta v's of about 16 mph (at 15 to 19 g), caused initial hyperextension of the necks and then hyperflexion on rebound. Five of the 6 cadavers sustained cervical injuries, none of which involved the spinal cord itself. Five of the 6 ruptured the anterior longitudinal ligament at C6,7 (clearly a hyperextension injury) and also sustained less severe C6,7 injuries to the vertebral bodies or to the intervertebral discs at these levels, some of which *may* be considered to have resulted from the rebound hyperflexion. Hyperextension injuries then are more severe than the hyperflexion injuries which result from rear end collision.

Typical hyperflexion injuries, such as tears of the posterior longitudinal ligament, of the interspinous ligaments or of the ligamentum flavum did not occur at all. It should also be noted that cadavers, as were used in this study, tend to exaggerate both the incidence and severity of injuries[3], perhaps because they lack active muscle support of the highly mobile cervical skeletal and ligamentous structures.

Partyka[18] reported an increase in "whiplash" injuries sustained by 3 point restrained occupants relative to unrestrained occupants (about a 30 percent increase for restrained occupants), as did a report by Larder et al[19] four years later, which referenced a relative increase in "neck sprains" of about 18 percent as seat belt usage in the U.K. increased from 26 percent to 93 percent.

Larder's study (as have others) also found that, for restrained occupants, these AIS 1 and lesser neck injuries:

1) occur without interior contact 2/3rds of the time,
2) occur more often in women than in men,
3) do not increase with increasing age,
4) are under-reported, because of delayed onset of symptoms,
5) occur often in crashes with only slight vehicle damage, and
6) had surprisingly protracted periods of disability: e.g., 40 percent had symptoms lasting in excess of a month and 8 percent had neck pain lasting longer than 6 months.

Because we are running into phrases such as "whiplash" injuries, and "neck sprains'' we'd best stop here and rinse this terminology in some sort of semantic laundry.

But first let us distinguish rear collisions into 2 categories, 1) the severe and fatal category — about 5 to 10 percent of all fatal car crashes we decided earlier in this chapter (and 3.5 percent in recent surveys) — and, 2) into the apparently trivial collisions which cause little or almost no damage to the vehicles but cause considerable neck injury and extensive disability to occupants of the largely undamaged cars.

The reason for the disparity and apparent paradoxic response between severe crashes with much vehicular damage causing either death or relatively minor neck injury, and modest crashes with little vehicular damage causing a lot of neck injuries (often with a lot of subsequent disability) is in understanding what each of these categories of rear collision does to the neck and in understanding what each of these accident categories means to occupant kinematics.

When a car is struck from the rear it is accelerated forward. An occupant of the car will be, to paraphrase Sir Isaac Newton, ''a body at rest that will tend to stay at rest,'' which is to say the occupant tries to stay put. But the occupant's seat back is attached to the car and is therefore thrust forward with the car, carrying the occupant's trunk with it. The head, unlike the trunk, is generally not resting against the seat back, and tries to stay put as the trunk is carried forward, causing hyperextension of the neck, which stays with the forward moving trunk at the lower end of the neck, and with the head (which tries to stay where it was) at the upper end of the neck.

Although I doubt that most of us are aware of it, car seat backs are remarkably flexible. When a seat back is bent backwards by the inertia of an occupant's upper body because the car was struck from the rear at a *low delta v*, the seat back will deform rearwards to an angle of something less than 60 degrees. The occupant's neck will thus be *hyperextended*, often thereby causing hyperextension injuries. When the seat back is bent back more than 60 degrees or so, (and it is bent to more than 60 degrees in *high delta v* rear impacts), the neck is put into *tension*[20], which is far less liable to damage its structures than is hyperextension. The net result of all of this is that the lower car collision damage rear impacts are more liable to cause significant neck injuries (because they put the neck into hyperextension) than are the high car collision damage rear impacts (which are more liable to put the neck in tension).

Now let's go on to briefly discuss such nasty terms as ''whiplash.''

Whiplash, Cervical Sprains, Strains and Other Soft Tissue Neck Injuries

In 1928, Dr. Harold E. Crow, reporting to the Western Orthopedic Association on 8 cases of neck injuries resulting from automobile crashes, first used the term "whiplash." He later (1963) was quoted as describing the use of the term as "unfortunate" in that he intended the term to be a description of motion, not as the name of a disease entity[21].

To others the name is unacceptable whether applied to an injury or mechanism of injury, for the cervical spine "is a relatively short-jointed structure, made up of separate rigid segments, with a ten pound weight at its end" and should not be compared to a whip, "which is long, unjointed, evenly flexible throughout its length, and has no weight on the end . . . The term to the honest is merely a bulwark behind which ignorance skulks; to the dishonest a mirage with which to confuse and delude[22]."

Because the term has been applied to describe: cervical sprains, cervical strains, flexion injuries, extension injuries, injuries in which elements of both hyperflexion and hyperextension are present, as well as: to describe different mechanisms of how cervical sprains and strains may be caused, to the effects of forward, lateral and rear collisions; it appears to have whatever meaning one claims for it.

I would be happier if the term went the way that I hope that other non-descriptive descriptors, such as "slipped disc" and "indigestion" as well as other, equally maliciously indefinite but colorful expressions would go, which is to say I wish they would go away, since they are misleading and vague at their very best.

Let's just say that what we're discussing is acceleration caused soft tissue cervical pathology that often persists.

How long does it persist? In 3 separate studies discussed by Macnab[23] a consistent 12 percent of patients sustaining "acceleration extension injuries of the cervical spine" (as Macnab chose to call it) went on to have significant impairment which interfered with their work and quality of life for a period of *years*. That is a remarkable finding to me.

After all, Partyka[18] tells us to expect some type of collision caused inertial force neck injury in more than 700,000 occupants each year, according to her analysis of the National Accident Sampling System. If 12 percent of these injuries go on to a significant impairment for a term of years, that's more than 80,000 of our citizens being impaired annually by cervical injuries that are miscalled "whiplash."

As to what specific pathology characterizes "acceleration extension injuries of the cervical spine," Macnab[23] reports anesthetized animal studies, including primate studies, which found tears of muscle, facet fractures, partial intervertebral disc separations and worse. Be again cautioned that, like cadavers, anesthetized animals do not have much muscle tone and support, and would be expected therefore to sustain injuries worse than would occur without anesthesia.

There is little doubt, in my mind at least, that cervical acceleration extension injuries can and do occur to car occupants in the absence of very much damage to the vehicle in which the occupant was located, and that about 10 percent of these injuries do go on to realize a chronic status from pathophysiologically based injuries. It should be noted however, that statistically this is still the exception and not the rule, (i.e., it is not more likely to occur than not occur) and that this applies nearly uniquely to the lower cervical spine, at C4-7.

ROLLOVER AND EJECTION

These subjects are often combined because rollover is the most common cause of ejection. Indeed, ejection is 10 to 15 times more usual in rollover[24].

Rollover

When we compare 1) *simple rollover* with 2) *collision-and-rollover* with 3) *non-rollover collision*, we find that the probability of *severe* injury is about 2 1/2 times as great in collision-and-rollover as compared to non-rollover collision. The probability of *severe* injury from simple rollover (without collision) is about 2 times that of simple (non-rollover) collision alone[25]. To restate the decreasing order of probable *severe* injury, it should read:

collision-and-rollover is worse than simple rollover, which is worse than simple collision

I used italics above to emphasize that we are dealing with *severe* injuries only. As far as I know, there are no studies which compare these events with regard to lesser injuries, especially in the absence of ejection as a factor.

Rollovers are deceptive events. Even observers that might be expected to be skilled observers, say a highway patrolman, will almost invariably report that the rollover vehicle did 3 to 5 or more full revolutions.

This is just so much nonsense. Studies which have included the number of quarter turns of rollover have shown that **90 percent of rollovers involve one full revolution (4 quarter turns) *or less***[24]. Some 67 percent of rollovers are a *half turn or less*. Between 1 and 2 full revolutions (4 to 7 quarter turns) represent less than 6 percent of rollovers, and so **only 1 of every 25 rollovers will do 8 or more quarter turns (2 full revolutions or more)**.

There is a strong tendency for rollover vehicles to do an even number of quarter turns because, as you might expect, rollover vehicles end up most often on either their wheels or their roofs[24].

You may also want to know that 4 of every 5 rollover vehicles travel less than 80 feet after the start of rollover[24].

While rollovers have a bad reputation, *in the absence of ejection* they do not seem that bad to me, at least as compared to say, a barrier impact.

Think about it. Would you rather give up your kinetic energy in say, 2 feet of crush that happens in a single blow or would you rather have a series of swats, each by itself of relatively low energy, albeit each swat comes at you from a different direction? If well restrained, I'd prefer the multiple low energy hits, although I have not found a good study of what the non-ejection total injuries would be for well restrained occupants at the same initial speed in barrier versus rollover collisions.

In the more than a few rollovers that I have dealt with, it appears that injuries either are lethal or very severe, say paraplegia, or are trivial. Rollovers seem to me to leave no middle ground for moderate injuries.

A recent (1991) characterization of rollover injuries[26] in data from the National Accident Sampling System (NASS) is especially helpful because it contains increased data on restrained occupants and because it is reported in terms of "harm," an index which better reflects disability rather than the more common Abbreviated Injury Scale (AIS). Their findings show that:

1) Most car rollovers are single vehicle crashes.
2) 97 percent of the rollovers are in roll, rather than pitch.
3) Rollovers result from higher travel speed and the outcome of the crash not surprisingly relates to the vehicle speed at the start of the crash/rollover.
4) In the 1988-89 NASS files, 48 percent of the rollover car occupants were restrained, and underwent only 22 percent of the "harm."
5) Head/face/neck injuries predominated both restrained and unrestrained occupants, with restrained occupants sustaining more neck injuries than unrestrained.
6) About 15 percent of the injuries to restrained occupants were due to the restraints themselves.

Ejection

When we consider ejection, it is of the utmost importance that we think of ejection and its related injuries in terms of whether the ejection resulted from collision-and-rollover, (pure) rollover, or (pure) collision.

There is a good deal of literature out there that lumps together all ejections regardless of the conditions that caused them. The statistics and conclusions that result therefore may well reflect that apples and oranges were counted together and we do not know how many of each there are.

An important, careful and useful study by Tonge and others[27] reported that "81 percent of those ejected received their major and fatal injuries within the vehicle before ejection, 13 percent outside the vehicle after ejection and 6 percent were killed by being crushed under an overturned vehicle." They also noted that 35 percent of the cases of ejection involved a pure rollover and in 45 percent of the cases there was a crash followed by rollover. (There was no information provided for the remaining 20 percent, but, presumably, the precedent condition was a pure crash followed by ejection.)

Roberts and Guenther[28] reevaluated the factors causing injury in ejections, reviewed the major related literature, and concluded that, for injuries sustained by ejected occupants:

1) most injuries are associated with vehicle interior impact,
2) most injuries occur either before or during ejection,
3) (for ejections following collision) "Ejection is more a measure of the violence of a collision than a measure of injury causation."
4) ejections mostly occur at high speed, involve young male drivers and occur disproportionately in a rural setting, all of which also characterizes fatal accidents whether or not ejection was a factor.

The issue of whether the amount of roof crush relates to occupant injury from rollover is a controversial issue in that there are a number of studies which report opposite conclusions, and the reader would be well advised to look to the latest reports for the latest opinions. At this time, I go with Orlowski et al[29] who, after a nice literature review of the subject, reported on some full scale tests, concluding (as have others) that "roof strength is not an important factor in the mechanics of head/neck injuries in rollover collisions for unrestrained occupants." Nor have I seen good evidence that roof crush would be an important causal factor of rollover head/neck injuries in restrained occupants.

Perhaps the way to wrap up the combined topics of rollover and ejection is to review a 1989 paper by Esterlitz[29], which studied risk of ejection death according to crash type and crash mode. She found that *single-vehicle crashes* (crash type) *with rollover* (crash mode) *had the highest increased risk of death due to ejection.* The risk increased about 8 times for the driver and was 7 times greater for the right front passenger.

SUMMARY

In this last chapter we have reviewed the patterns of injury for crashes and found that frontal, lateral and rear crashes indeed have injury patterns that typify them.

Frontal collisions were found most often to be offset to one side or the other, with *left frontal collisions being the most common.* The preponderance of left-sidedness of frontal collisions may more rationally account for whatever differences exist between lower limb injuries of the driver and right front passenger than many other theories (i.e., opinions) that so abundantly have been propounded without any basis at all.

Lateral collisions were found to have vehicle intrusion as a major injury producing event. Lateral collisions were also found to suffer from faults of current 3-point seat belt restraints: first, that the lap belt portion holds the occupant in location as the intruding vehicle tries to occupy the same location, and second, that the upper diagonal portion of the 3-point restraint does not restrain the occupant on the far side of the side struck vehicle.

Rear collisions were found to be lightly represented as a cause of death and heavily overrepresented as a cause of disability.

Rollover crashes were found to be modified by whether or not the rollover was preceded by a collision, since ejections from collisions or from collisions followed by rollovers have most injuries occurring within the vehicle, prior to ejection. It is often less clear as to where injuries occurred in simple rollovers without prior collisions, whether they occurred within the vehicle during rollover or whether they occurred outside of the vehicle, after ejection.

BIBLIOGRAPHY

1. Otte, D., von Rheinbaben, H. and H. Zwipp: Biomechanics of injuries to the foot and ankle joint of car drivers and improvements for an optimal car floor development. *SAE* paper 922514, 1992.
2. Gloyns, P.F., Hayes, H.R.M., Rattenbury, S.J., Thomas, P.D., Mills, H.C. and D.K. Griffiths: Lower limb injuries to car occupants in frontal impacts. *Proc IRCOBI Conf*, p. 105, 1979.
3. Kallieris, D., Mellander, H., Schmidt, G., Barz, J. and R. Mattern: Comparison between frontal impact tests with cadavers and dummies in a simulated true car restrained environment. *SAE* paper 821170, 1982.
4. Dalmotas, D.J.: Mechanisms of injury to vehicle occupants restrained by three-point seat belts. *SAE* paper 801311, 1980.
5. Dance, M. and B. Enserink: Safety performance evaluation of seat belt retractors. *SAE* paper 790680, 1979.
6. Gloyns, P.F., Rattenbury, S.J., Rivlin, A.Z., Hayes, H.R.M., Hanstead, J.K. and S. Proctor: Steering wheel induced head and facial injuries amongst drivers restrained by seat belts. *Proc IRCOBI Conf*, p. 30, 1981.
7. Malliaris, A.C., Hitchcock, R. and M. Hansen: Harm causation and ranking in car crashes. *SAE* paper 850090, 1985.
8. Faerber, E.: Interaction of car passengers in frontal, side and rear collisions. *SAE* paper 821167, 1982.
9. Lestina, D.C., Gloyns, P.F. and S.J. Rattenbury: Fatally injured occupants in side impact crashes. *IIHS*, 1990.
10. Careme, L.M.M.: Occupant kinematics and injury causation in side impacts— field accident experience. *SAE* paper 910316, 1991.
11. Mills, P.J. and C.A. Hobbs: The probability of injury to car occupants in frontal and side impacts. *SAE* paper 841652, 1984.
12. Daniel, R.P.: Biomechanical design considerations for side impact. *SAE* paper 890386, 1989.
13. Data Link, Inc., 1989/1990 statistics, quoted in Viano, D.C.: Influence of seatback angle on occupant dynamics in simulated rear-end impacts. *SAE* paper 922521, 1992.
14. Huelke, D.F. and J.C. Marsh: Analysis of rear-end accident factors and injury patterns. *Proc 18th Ann Conf AAAM*, 1974.
15. Tarriere, C.: Pathophysiology and mechanisms — neck injury. In: *Head and Neck Injury Criteria*, U.S. Govt. Printing Office, Washington, D.C.,

March, 1981.

16. Lovsund, P., Nygren, A., Salen, B. and C. Tingvall: Neck injuries in rear end collisions among front and rear seat occupants. *Proc IRCOBI Conf*, p. 319, 1988.

17. Jones, A.M., Bean, S.P. and E.S. Sweeney: Injuries to cadavers resulting from experimental rear impact. *J Forensic Sci, 23*:730, 1978.

18. Partyka, S.: Whiplash and other inertial force neck injuries in traffic accidents. *National Center for Statistics and Analysis*, NHTSA, DOT, Washington, D.C., 1981, and in DOT-HS-806 403, 1983.

19. Larder, D.R., Twiss, M.K. and G.M. Mackay: Neck injury to car occupants using seat belts. *Proc 29th Ann Conf AAAM*, p. 153, 1985.

20. Viano, D.C.: Influence of seatback angle on occupant dynamics in simulated rear-end impacts. *SAE* paper 922521, 1992.

21. Curran, W.J. and N.L. Chayet: *Trauma and the Automobile.* Anderson, Cincinnati, 1966.

22. Bosworth, D.: Editorial. *J Bone Joint Surg 41-A*:16, 1959.

23. Macnab, I.: Acceleration extension injuries of the cervical spine. In Rothman, R.H. and F.A. Simeone: *The Spine.* 2nd ed., Saunders, Philadelphia, 1982, vol II, pp. 647-660.

24. McGuigan, R. and N. Bondy: A descriptive study of rollover crashes. In NHTSA, *DOT HS-805-883*, 1981.

25. Najjar, D.: The truth about rollovers. *ibid.*

26. Digges, K.H., Malliaris, A.C., Ommaya, A.K. and A.J. McLean: Characterization of rollover casualties. *Proc IRCOBI Conf*, p. 309, 1991.

27. Tonge, J.I., O'Reilly, M.J.J., Davison, A. and N.G. Johnston: Traffic crash fatalities. Injury patterns and other factors. *Med J Aust 2*:5, 1972.

28. Roberts, V.L. and D.A. Guenther: Ejection versus injury: A reevaluation. *Proc 3rd Canad Multidiscip Road Safety Conf*, 1984.

29. Orlowski, K.F., Bundorf, R.T. and E.A. Moffat: Rollover crash tests — the influence of roof strength on injury mechanics. *SAE* paper 651734, 1985.

30. Esterlitz, J.R.: Relative risk of death from ejection by crash type and crash mode. *Accid Anal Prev 21*:459, 1989.